Educating Doctors' Senses Through the Medical Humanities

Educating Doctors' Senses Through the Medical Humanities: "How Do I Look?" uses the medical diagnostic method to identify a chronic symptom in medical culture: the unintentional production of insensibility through compulsory mis-education. This book identifies the symptom and its origins and offers an intervention: deliberate and planned education of sensibility through the introduction of medical humanities to the core undergraduate medicine and surgery curriculum.

To change medical culture is an enormous challenge, and this book sets out how to do this by answering the following questions:

- How has a compulsory mis-education for insensibility developed in medical culture and medical education?
- How is sensibility capital generated, who 'owns' it and how is it distributed, mal-distributed and re-distributed? What is the place of resistance (or 'dissensus') in this process?
- How can the symptom of a 'developed' insensibility be addressed pedagogically through introduction of the medical humanities as core and integrated curriculum provision?
- How can both the identity constructions of doctors and doctor–patient relationships be tied up with education for sensibility?
- How can artists work with clinicians, through the medical humanities in medical education, to better educate sensibility?

The book will be of interest to all medical educators and clinicians, including those health and social care professionals outside of medicine who work with doctors.

Alan Bleakley is Emeritus Professor at the University of Plymouth's Peninsula School of Medicine and Dentistry, UK.

Routledge Advances in the Medical Humanities

For more information about this series visit: www.routledge.com/ Routledge-Advances-in-the-Medical-Humanities/book-series/RAMH

Educating Doctors' Senses Through the Medical Humanities

"How Do I Look?"

Alan Bleakley

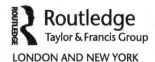

Routledge
Taylor & Francis Group

LONDON AND NEW YORK

First published 2020 by Routledge

2 Park Square, Milton Park, Abingdon, Oxon OX14 4RN
605 Third Avenue, New York, NY 10017

Routledge is an imprint of the Taylor & Francis Group, an informa business

First issud in paperback 2021

British Library Cataloguing-in-Publication Data
A catalogue record for this book is available from the British Library

Library of Congress Cataloging-in-Publication Data
Names: Bleakley, Alan (Alan Douglas), author.
Title: Educating doctors' senses through the medical humanities : "How do I look?" / Alan Bleakley.
Description: Abingdon, Oxon ; New York, NY : Routledge, 2020. | Includes bibliographical references and index.
Identifiers: LCCN 2019049108 (print) | LCCN 2019049109 (ebook)
Subjects: MESH: Education, Medical—methods | Humanities—education | Sensation | Philosophy, Medical
Classification: LCC R737 (print) | LCC R737 (ebook) | NLM W 18 | DDC 610.71/1—dc23
LC record available at https://lccn.loc.gov/2019049108
LC ebook record available at https://lccn.loc.gov/2019049109

ISBN: 978-0-367-20248-4 (hbk)
ISBN: 978-1-03-217520-1 (pbk)
DOI: 10.4324/9780429260438

Typeset in Times New Roman
by codeMantra

Dedicated to my wife Sue, who woke up my senses; and to my loving family: Phaedra, Brioney, Sam, Jonty, Sandy, Issy, Lola, Amelie and Ruben.

Contents

Foreword

From joyfully holding a slippery, salty newborn, listening to the humdrum lub-dub of the heart or recoiling from a fungating tumour, medicine is a practice of the senses through an educated immersion in a sensory world, following Maurice Merleau-Ponty's (1945/1962: 94) observation that "The body is the vehicle of being in the world, and having a body is, for a creature, to be intervolved in a definite environment, to identify oneself with certain projects and be continually committed to them". Sight, smell, sound and touch are fundamental tools of physicianship. Yet the experiential nature of these sensory skills is suppressed in contemporary medical education, resulting in a numbing of both the senses and the sensitivities of clinicians. The consequences are costly for both patients and doctors. For patients, an increased reliance on technology over *techne* or craft risks over-diagnoses, mis-diagnoses and inappropriate uses of medications. Physicians are more likely to experience emotional detachment, empathy decline and become susceptible to burnout or dysfunctional behaviour.

In this provocative and challenging book, Alan Bleakley argues that sedating the senses has resulted in an erosion of the moral compass of medicine. The mis-education of insensibility dehumanises and colonises medical identity by systematically shutting down the doctor's fundamental means of experiencing the world – the body. There is a moral and political imperative to change how we desensitise and disavow the embodied experiences of becoming a physician. Developing recurrent themes of his work, Bleakley calls for the democratisation of medical education and a flattening of power structures to more consciously attend to the senses. His solution is a more equitable education in the arts, where artist and clinician co-educate, learning with and from each other. In this way, humanities provoke and enliven, salve and save, enabling the medical profession to boldly confront its corporeal reality.

In engaging and wide-ranging prose, this book brings the senses to our attention, helping the reader to experience the cornucopia of sensory knowledge that is medical practice. Chapters open with anecdotes set in clinical contexts, which invite us to ponder a particular sense in health care. For practical reasons, the text is separated into chapters attentive to the different senses, but a central message is the joined-up nature of the senses as a system, and how as individuals our senses are linked with those of our fellow humans. Our senses extend beyond the individual, entwined in the environment and the interconnectedness of the human condition, a move from 'I am in my body' to 'I am my body', and more – 'I am my body in the world'. The text draws on a breadth of literature, evidencing the significance and potential of each sense. Auto-ethnography, observational data and case studies from wide-spanning sources are woven together to substantiate the thesis in an enticing format, making the text a valuable resource for a broader readership beyond the medical education community.

Yet, for those of you hoping for a soothing read, beware. This book will make you squirm. You may even be repelled. For, as Bleakley invites us to consider the vibrant sensory nature of an embodied medical practice, he draws on aesthetics not as a form of sensory relaxation but to reveal the abject nature of medical education. Superficially, Bleakley rouses us by describing the physical excreta of human suffering – vomit, faeces, pus and normally unarticulated aspects of experiencing illness. But exposing deeper strata, he playfully deconstructs false idols of present-day education such as simulation by contrasting the messy swill and sluicing of sickness with an education which trains with plasticized, genderless, standardized dolls, housed in odourless clinical skills laboratories.

Applying his psychoanalytic training, Bleakley pins medical education to the psychologist's couch, using Freud and Lacan to examine how formative experiences in medical education suppress innately human sensory responses, returning in a distorted form as harmful and dysfunctional identity formation. Without our senses, in denying the body-subject (ibid), we are unable to make 'sense' of the material world, where cognitive processing in isolation congeals and concretizes experience into abstracted entities. Drawing on Julia Kristeva's work on the abject, a case is built that medical education has failed to reconcile the disgusting with the sensitive, resulting in emotional fracture and disembodied learning. To experience beauty, we must reconcile the base. To be sensitive, we must burrow into the horror of suffering and stare the tumour in the eye, touch its rugged splendour with hand and mind while fully respecting the suffering patient. This deeper engagement with the body is explored by performance artists such as Martin O'Brien and ORLAN, artistry that demands by physically confronting us with the body as 'living maps of power and identity' (Haraway 1994).

This is a volume born of emancipatory vigilance. To re-humanise medicine and promote its tender-minded values, we are invited to radically reflect on the political consequences of sensory subjugation which reinforce a normative, hegemonic privileging of the body, moulding and crafting physicians' and patients' bodies as the patina of medical culture, replicated through the generations. Bleakley challenges the docile body of medical education by drawing attention to the interdependent dialectics of the sensory body, power and identity. At a time when medical education is calling for

increased diversity, it is essential that this is not just levied at socially con-
structed notions of power but rooted in the marrow, and for change to happen, the vulnerable flesh of patients and learners needs to be acknowledged
and liberated.

Dr Martina Ann Kelly
Associate Professor and Director of Undergraduate
Family Medicine, Cumming School of Medicine,
University of Calgary; family medicine physician.

Introduction

Medicine's push–pull relations with the senses

A paradoxical disengagement from the body runs deep in medicine and has distinct historical roots. While it deals with bodies, modern medicine can be described as disembodied. How did this come about? Through dissection and subsequent careful archiving in production of lavish anatomical atlases, the Flemish physician and anatomist Andreas Vesalius (1514–1564) introduced an instrumental way of looking at the body that stripped away sentiment or feeling to be replaced by an objective eye. The body was not just dismembered in being reduced to its component parts but also disembodied where treated as a machine. Wonder now resided in the body's anatomised instrumental efficiency in a 'naming of parts' and not in its fleshy, sensory surprise. The body was both spectacularised and stylised through the anatomy text. In Vesalius's wake, René Descartes (1596–1650) argued that our only certainty is the thinking 'I', where body and mind are conveniently separated, and body is subservient to mind. The Cartesian says 'I am *in* my body', where the phenomenologist says 'I *am* my body' (Young 1989).

Disembodied practices continue to haunt medicine. For most medical students in North America and Africa, the first 'patient' they meet is a cadaver (the strangest form of disembodied medicine because there are no words or exchanges to flesh out meanings between the 'first patient' and the novice medical student). A second 'patient' is a hard plastic, silicon and latex bells-and-whistles manikin used in simulation learning for clinical and communication skills. More, it is white and male ('SimMan'). The medical student then swings between the extremes of the abject (deep emotional engagement through disgust in meeting a preserved corpse) and the object (emotional suspension in meeting the odourless plastic model). A third patient is at last flesh and blood and in a hospital bed, but possibly protected from 'warm' hands-on physical examination, supplanted by 'cold' investigative and diagnostic technologies. Where these technologies might offer more accurate diagnostic capacity, 'hands-on' examinations serve the crucial purpose of creating a bond with the patient. Even with hands-on contact, the patient, however, may be objectified as a disease classification, a diagnostic marker.

Such disembodied pedagogies can lead to production of insensibility and insensitivity. By 'sensibility', I mean primarily the biological dictionary (*Shorter Oxford English Dictionary*) definition: "sensitivity to sensory stimuli", which includes "sensory discrimination" (key to clinical acumen). This extends to the wider definition of "the quality of being able to appreciate and respond to complex emotional or aesthetic influences" (key to communication with patients and colleagues). While 'sensibility' and 'sensitivity' are often used interchangeably, I use the former as oriented particularly to sense perception and awareness of embodiment, where the latter is oriented to quality in relationship and emotional or affective response. Production of both insensibility and insensitivity is an unintended consequence of a medical education, but there is also an intended consequence, where medical students are protected from getting too close emotionally to their patients for fear of affective overload or invasion clouding rational judgement. This typically results in the development of a professional persona, a distancing or emotional insulation. Medicine at this point becomes performative. An identity construction describing 'professionalism' (a 'proto-professionalism') is seeded, paralleling that of 'medical trainee'. Working with SimMan to learn clinical skills in simulation settings requires another kind of performativity – pretence that this plastic model is indeed a flesh and blood person who is being resuscitated.

A creeping disembodiment of medical practice has led clinicians and medical educators such as Martina Kelly (Kelly et al. 2019) to call for developing 'body pedagogics' – a medical education grounded in the senses. Shilling (2017: 1205) describes body pedagogics as "an embodied approach to the transmission and acquisition of ... culturally structured practices". In medicine, for example, this refers to the transmission and interpretation of medical knowledge, practices and values as these engage both material culture and bodily activities. Central to this is the shaping or crafting of an embodied identity or subjectivity – again, not 'I am in my body', but 'I am my body' and 'I perform my body'.

In medicine, a tradition of disembodied practice has been countered historically by instances of formal body engagement, for example, in the development of palpation, percussion and auscultation as hands-on diagnostic techniques, discussed in depth in later chapters. The Austrian physician Leopold Auenbrugger (1722–1809), who codified percussing the body as a diagnostic technique, restored touch and embodiment to an intellectual medicine dominated by the Vesalian anatomical tradition and Cartesian legacy. The introduction of mediate auscultation by René Laennec (1781–1826), the inventor of the stethoscope, reinforced this embrace of an embodied medicine (see Chapter 4).

Yet the education of the senses remains poorly conceived and disorganised in undergraduate medical education curricula today, where learning medicine is anchored in the reproduction of the medical gaze established as a dominant discourse for over two centuries. Michel Foucault's (1976) classic account of the birth of modern medicine argues that the yoking of 'the birth of the clinic' as a teaching space (the teaching hospital) with the anatomy laboratory (cadaver dissection) nourished the development of a distinct 'medical perception'. This is popularly termed the medical 'gaze' (*regard*), masculinised where it embraces ocular 'penetration' and objectification of the body as a gesture of power of doctor over patient.

In *Dissection: Photographs of a Rite of Passage in American Medicine 1880–1930*, John Harley Warner and James Edmonson (2009) recount extreme examples of modern medical perception. White, mostly male, medical students – exuding arrogance – are shown posing with human cadavers and skeletons, continuing a form of (an)aesthetic stylisation introduced by Vesalius. The cadavers and skeletons are mostly African American persons and obtained by dubious means – stolen from graves or claimed by the state.

The authors argue that the photographs show an intimacy between medical students and 'their' cadavers lost after the 1930s as "a new era of objectivity and detachment entered medical education, ending the earlier emotional attachment to the dissection process" (Lerner 2009: unpaginated). However, this is a rather perverse 'intimacy', where, shockingly, "Some of the dissection images contain racist inscriptions, such as 'Sliced Nigger', from the Wake Forest School of Medicine; and 'All Coons Smell Alike to Us', from the College of Physicians and Surgeons of Baltimore" (ibid). As the Introduction by Lerner (in Werner and Edmonson 2006) suggests,

> Every medical school … should get a hold of the images in this remarkable volume and show them to incoming students before they set foot in an anatomy lab. The mistakes of their predecessors might impart a needed dose of humility.

It can be argued that modern anatomy learning from cadaver dissection in North American and European medical schools in particular has then been about establishing and reinforcing the penetrative medical gaze through a ritual initiation in the name of white, male imperialism and heroic individualism. Lingering, institutionalised superiority, racism and sexism still infect medicine where it continues to refuse democracy, feminising and tenderminded (optimistic, idealistic) rather than tough-minded (pessimistic and cynical) values.

An embodied, or sense-based, medicine could restore feminine values and practices of sensibility and sensitivity that have been lost to an education of insensibility and insensitivity based on the medical gaze. Indeed, borrowing from Paul Goodman (1964) – who first coined the term to describe misguided compulsory schooling – I suggest that this is a "compulsory miseducation" of insensibility and insensitivity. Goodman noted a disjunction between what pupils learn and preparation to become an engaged and critically reflexive citizen.

Such an individualistic medical gaze has been displaced in an era in which the gaze's destiny is collaborative (authentic patient-centredness and inter-professionalism), nourishing (feminine?) and embodied (Bleakley and Bligh 2009). An epistemic rupture is promised in medicine and medical education in which a collaborative process restores an educated sensibility (for clinical acumen) and sensitivity (for patient and colleague communication) to medicine. *This book sets out an argument and a method for reconceptualising the education of the senses in undergraduate medical education in particular, through critical incorporation of the medical humanities.*

Culture's sensory paradox

The paradox that medicine seeks to educate the senses at the same time as it encourages sensory dulling resonates with a wider cultural phenomenon. Where modernism paradoxically introduced sensory refinements as it increased sensory overload, this was paralleled by developments in anaesthesia involving nitrous oxide, chloroform and ether (Buck-Morss 1992). Globally, a large array of anxiolytic drugs is now used not to enhance perception but to dull the senses in the face of escalating levels of anxiety generated culturally (Campbell 2017).

Such public anxiety – an anomie, or sense of loss of a moral compass – is described by Cressida Heyes (2020) as an "anaesthetics of existence". She calls for an embodied (and feminised) "aesthetics of existence". Heyes points to the tradition of 20th-century cultural studies literature (particularly the work of Walter Benjamin) in suggesting that the modern human sensorium is traumatised (in the wake of two world wars, the nuclear cold war and the rise of mass consumerism) and then de-sensitises as a response to environmental sensory overload. We readily slip out of our embodied states to protect ourselves from traumatic sensory overload – and this seems like an immediate explanation for why medicine promises an education of the senses for improving clinical acumen or close noticing, but delivers insensibility and insensitivity.

Continuing production of insensibility and insensitivity through medical education is evidenced in

1   Relatively high levels of misdiagnoses (Graber and Berner 2008; Newman-Toker and Pronovost 2009; Newman-Toker 2014) and medical errors (Bleakley 2014).
2   An increasingly over-determined medicine that includes over-diagnosing and over-prescribing (Welch et al. 2011). This is partly in response to an increased threat of patient litigation for medical error, but is also grounded in fear of failure.
3   Empathy decline, emotional detachment and insulation and creeping cynicism in later years medical students (Eikeland et al. 2014; Peng et al. 2018).
4   Doctors' poor self-care. While doctors' health is clearly affected by structural conditions such as long hours under emotional duress, there is also a longstanding cultural norm of self-inflicted exhaustion (heroic invincibility) and denial of symptom (Peterkin and Bleakley 2017).

Stemming the disembodiment of medicine

The surgical education work of Roger Kneebone (2019) shows how learning embodied practice can be intensified and accelerated through the arts and crafts and the work of laboratory scientists (Kneebone et al. 2018). Kneebone has worked as a surgeon and a general practitioner, and is a renowned surgical educator. His vision of a common connecting web of sensory capabilities between previously unconnected practices is matched by his tireless efforts to engage those practitioners in mutual mapping and comparison of bodily pedagogies that are often brought in turn to public engagement forums.

For example, tailors sew and so do surgeons – what can they learn from each other about eye–hand coordination? Laboratory scientists, in preparing samples, measuring, pouring, comparing and so on develop rhythms to their work and 'haptic knowledge' that crafts experts also share, where "Laboratory knowing takes place at the intersection between materials, tools and a researcher's body. Its rhythms differ from those of simply absorbing facts" (ibid: 188). Kneebone and colleagues ask: "how people steeped in artistic skills might help to close this 'haptic gap', the deficit in skills of touch and object manipulation" (ibid). Performers and craftspeople can collaborate with scientists to ratchet up performance levels, insight and creative possibilities. For example, how experts use their senses reveals

> striking similarities between the observational skills of an entomologist and an analytical chemist; the dexterity of a jeweller and a microsurgeon; the bodily awareness of a dancer and a space scientist; and the creative skills of a scientific glassblower, a reconstructive surgeon, a potter and a chef (ibid).

Kneebone has also addressed the criticism that learning clinical skills *in vitro* – as simulation – rather than *in vivo*, largely for purposes of patient safety, cultivates insensibility. Using more realistic body models such as simulated flesh wounds developed by expert make-up artists who normally work in television and, importantly, creating intensive but low-cost environments and scripted scenarios for practice, where surgical teamwork is treated as performance, Kneebone addresses central concerns about insensibility as an unintended consequence of simulated learning. Such work on "immersive, distributed simulation" can engage those beyond clinical 'insiders', such as the general public, managers, policymakers and commissioners (Weldon et al. 2019).

At Maastricht University in the Netherlands, an interdisciplinary research group echoes Kneebone's desire to better understand commonalities across practices engaged in sensory education. They focus upon one sensory modality – sound (with some reference to touch). The 'Sonic Skills' project (Bijsterveld 2018) describes 'Listening for Knowledge in Science, Medicine and Engineering'. It analyses how a variety of scientists, including doctors, develop the art of listening as a basis to their work, described as 'sensory practices' that address 'embodied representations' (for doctors, 'symptom presentations'). Importantly, the researchers in this project allow descriptors such as 'wonder' and 'awe' to describe sonic practices, which are more at home in the arts than in science and technology.

Anthropologists such as Tim Ingold (1999, 2000), studying the gaining of craft expertise across cultures, refer to 'enskillment' as a process of perceptual attunement through embedding in an ecology. Learning environments, such as wards in hospitals, offer specific ecologies affording specific patterns shaping embodied practices, where we must go beyond the solipsistic individual (an ego-logic) to an eco-logical perspective that emphasises how environmental cues come to shape perception or 'educate attention'. Junior learners – medical students and junior doctors – adapt to habitats such as hospital wards, morbidity and mortality meetings and surgical theatres through close observation of 'old hands', even down to postures, proxemics, haptics, gestures and voice tones, expressed within an idiosyncratic local climate of lore and rules. They note how their seniors use their senses and follow suit, as their learning is scaffolded around a specialty's house of sensing until they are allowed to look in through the windows and finally enter via a door. Medicine, as this book shows, has its own idiosyncratic cultural pathways for developing the senses.

Such a traditional apprenticeship model – an initiation into a community of practice as absorption of habits – has largely characterised undergraduate medical education until relatively recently (Bleakley et al. 2011; Bleakley 2014; Engeström 2019). Clinical practice involving temporary or 'liquid' inter-professional teams demands now that younger doctors think on their feet more and are able to tolerate high levels of ambiguity. There is a rapid shift from traditional models of apprenticeship requiring a will-to-stability and emphasising an individual locus of expertise to collaborative expertise and learning for change. Medical education must lead students to identity constructions that embrace 'possibility knowledge' and innovation as agents of change. This requires a shift in bodily sense from isolated body (the ego-logical) to social and incorporated body (the eco-logical). A revolution in perception is required, demanding new approaches in medical education informed by the medical humanities.

Eco-logical vs ego-logical perception

Constance Classen's (2014) edited six volumes of *A Cultural History of the Senses* provide multiple examples of how the senses are entrained differently by cultures through history, and, for example, Kathryn Geurts's (2003) *Culture and the Senses: Bodily Ways of Knowing in an African Community* reminds us of cultural biases in sense education and embodied practices, such as the ocular-centricity of Western culture. Geurts's anthropological work describes the sensorium of Anlo-Ewe-speaking people in southeastern Ghana. Here, the western 'five senses' model makes little sense, where this community takes 'balance' as the dominant sense. This runs through literal balance (baskets on the head, carrying infants, standing, squatting, moving) to metaphors of balance, to psychological states of balance as perceptual frames, or ways of understanding and appreciating the world. This is the embodied work of 'making sense'.

The Anlo use *seselelame* (literally 'feel-feel-at-flesh-inside' – the closest western thinking might come to this is 'kinaesthesia', or proprioception and interoception) to describe a range of sensory experiences, including an approximation of what Heidegger referred to as 'indwelling' – an embodied being-in-the-world. This can be conceived as a consciousness *from* the body (a tacit knowing), rather than a consciousness *of* the body. As we think of a 'sense of foreboding' (an embodied metaphor), so the Anlo might see this as a glimpse into the future by 'leaning in' to it. Importantly, there is no mind–body dualism in the Anlo imagination. A lesson we can draw from this is that medical specialties tend to privilege differing senses and so we can think anthropologically about this in terms of translation across specialties of sense connoisseurship, challenging stereotyping. For example, how can the ocular sense modality preferences and biases of ophthalmology or radiology converse with the listening modality privileged in audiology or respiratory medicine?

To return to eco-logical rather than ego-logical perceptions (explored in more depth in Chapter 1), we don't choose to sense as an inward-to-outward process; rather, the environment affords patterns that shape our sensing. Nor are we static receivers of stimuli; rather, we move through environments as we are folded into them. The perceptual psychologist James J Gibson (1950) championed this view, where Tim Ingold (2000: 3) offers an elegant summary:

> Perception, Gibson argued, is not the achievement of a mind in a body, but of the organism as a whole in its environment, and is tantamount to the organism's own exploratory movement through the world. If mind is anywhere, then, it is not 'inside the head' rather than 'out there' in the world. To the contrary, it is immanent in the network of sensory pathways that are set up by virtue of the perceiver's immersion in his or her environment.

Learning can be thought of as meaningful inherence, or again 'indwelling'. Immersion is an event without any necessary meaning or implication. Learning occurs when an event becomes an experience, or the environment affords a pattern for insight. For example, Sarah Maslen's (2015) fieldwork describes how medical students are taught to turn ambient and relatively meaningless body sounds into meaningful patterns as a diagnostic skill, where the 'raw' sense of hearing initially affords unmediated knowledge. Students 'get' mediate auscultation using the stethoscope under tutelage, particularly listening to heart or lung sounds, as they stop thinking about searching for sounds during a physical examination and immerse themselves in sound as an ecological perception. This requires suspension of misdirected effort on the part of the student to relax into what is being pointed out by the patient or expert tutor as an education of attention.

In order to pick out a figure against an ambient sound background, the tutor scaffolds the learning through artful description, often drawing on metaphor (as likeness), as 'sonic alignment' (Vannini et al. 2010; Rice 2013) (see Chapter 5). Here, from Maslen's (2015) ethnographic account, we see how the students' classroom-based anatomical knowledge can be triangulated with direct clinical experience shaped by medical-historical-lore imagery and metaphor (Bleakley 2018) to produce meaning. A tutor explains to Maslen (2015: 61) what would also be explained to students early in clinical exposure about the beat of a normal heart:

> The first heart sound is generated by the mitral and tricuspid valves closing. During systole, where the heart contracts and expels blood from the left and right ventricles, that (sound) is associated with the closing of the mitral and tricuspid valves, which stop blood flowing into the ventricles at the same time from the atria. As they close that causes 'lub', and blood is expelled from the heart, and then at the end of systole or the contraction of the ventricles, the aortic and pulmonary valves close, and that gives the 'dub'.

I would extend Maslen's analysis to include students discussing that the 'lub-dub' (or 'lub-dup') of the heart is the basis for Shakespearean iambic pentameter, or five beats to a line. As in the word 'remark' the first syllable (re) is unstressed, the second (mark) is stressed, the whole constituting one 'beat'. Five of these beats form a line ('Lub-dup/lub-dup/lub-dup/lub-dup/lub-dup'), as "But, soft!/what light/through yon/der win/dow breaks?" (Shakespeare's *Romeo and Juliet*).

In Maslen's fieldwork, another heart sound – 'lub-di-dub' – was described as "like the spinnaker on a yacht" (the sound produced when the spinnaker sail fills with wind and balloons) (admittedly not much help if you don't sail), and a further heart sound as "like (the water from) a hose directly hitting against a bucket" (ibid: 63). We then have triangulation between (i) anatomical theory and knowledge, (ii) sensory experience (listening to the heart) and (iii) a metaphor or likeness (simile) that may or may not be in the student's experience. Thus, mind, body and imagination are simultaneously engaged.

Returning to Ingold's 'enskillment' model, while properly giving credibility to the embodiment of learning, this model still privileges the individual – again, an ego-logical model. We need to view enskillment as 'extended' and collaborative – an eco-logical model – with mutual scaffolding of learning amongst learners themselves as well as tutor-to-learner, extending to cultural artefacts.

Commentators on embodied practices can make too much of the differences between cognitions and actions, merely returning us to Cartesian dilemmas. Bodily events occur at differing scales. Thus, without resorting to reductionism, a broad and meaningful gesture is also a muscular and skeletal movement, a movement of blood and chemicals, a flexing of cell walls, mitochondria moving along actin tracks within the cell and, at the level of the brain, chemical tides and electrical impulses, pulses and storms. Our unit of analysis can change, but our inquiring paradigm of activity remains consistent. Phenomenology can be neurology without reduction. Scaling is not reductionism (Wiens 1989) – repeating patterns or fractals occur at differing levels in dynamic, complex, adaptive systems (www.patternthinking. com/repeating-patterns.html).

This book then brings to medical education – through the media of the medical humanities, as we shall see in subsequent chapters – a novel approach to educating sensibility and sensitivity. The first chapter makes a case for scaling – considering the senses as a complex system, where later chapters, for convenience, consider the familiar five senses. Chapter 2 expands the idea that medical students, promised a particular education of the senses, can actually receive a miseducation to include sensory insult, particularly in learning anatomy through cadaver dissection. The final Chapter 9 expands on a theme running throughout the book – that education of the senses in medicine is also a form of identity construction, one of 'becoming' a doctor and professional. This requires management of identity as performance.

Radical and innovative curriculum interventions are needed to foster democratic habits, feminisation and tender-mindedness to counter a miseducation of the senses. This calls for a thoughtful development of the medical humanities as core and integrated provision where the curriculum serves aesthetic, ethical and political purposes as well as the instrumental. Those interested in medical pedagogy can draw on this account of body pedagogics to review curriculum provision. I do not provide a formal curriculum map, but the ensuing chapters present a wealth of examples that can readily be translated into pedagogical activities.

1 Medicine making sense

The senses as a system

Transforming a burden, shaping doctors

An article in *The New York Times* recounts how dealing with patients close to death on a day-to-day basis began to take its toll (Puri 2019: unpaginated). The palliative care doctor Sunita Puri struggled with "how to doctor patients I knew I would lose", as he grew "progressively more anxious, and occasionally despondent … more withdrawn, less punctual and occasionally distracted". Puri's numbing of feelings, creeping anxiety and foggy depression are also the most common symptoms shown by doctors who over-identify with patients and are exhausted as a consequence. Further, the health care system can alienate, grinding one down. And it can create anomie where it appears that you are working in a culture providing little moral guidance, or one that has lost its own moral compass.

For the few, this numbing can rapidly tumble into burnout (Peterkin and Bleakley 2017), an unfortunate descriptor for what is better compared to cold ashes. For the many, in order to function on a daily basis such emotional perturbations are psychologically 'managed': repressed, projected, or sublimated, only to return in a distorted form as disillusionment, bitterness and exhaustion. Here, a switch to part-time work and/or early retirement may be the only way to deal with this burden of negative affect. Puri himself was tipped particularly, he says, by not understanding "why death had come for a 35-year-old mother of three with a rare cancer", and "why a marathon runner was dying after a sudden heart attack when he had been a *marathon runner*".

When his "sadness grew stronger", Puri was warned by colleagues that, in general, doctors do not look after themselves well, and he should try a relaxation technique or psychotherapeutic intervention. However, "massages, therapy, hiking and meditating under the shade of Marin County redwoods" did not help him. What did help – indeed was transformative – was a chance visit to a Vietnamese Buddhist temple near the hospital where he worked. Here, a group of Tibetan monks were "hunched over a table" creating a sand mandala – an intricate, coloured geometric flower 'painting' made by collaborative, cumulative and careful pouring of small amounts of sand.

This meticulous creation took many days to complete, but once finished and serenely contemplated, Puri was shocked that one of the monks took a brush to the work and, without remorse, quickly swept the sand into bags. As Puri notes, "the hands that created it were content to let it go". Buddhism teaches us to accept that all is change.

This lesson on impermanence – clearly appropriate to end of life care – had a lasting effect on Puri. In contrast to interventions from medical education, psychotherapy and mindfulness, a visual and performative art form and spiritual practice – a "painstakingly crafted mandala ... ablaze with colour" – mediated how Puri could "doctor my dying patients differently". He would still feel compassion for patients but "didn't leave work ... consumed with grief, withdrawn and disengaged". This lesson on impermanence then transformed not only Puri's care of his patients but also his growing existential angst and 'bad faith' in coming to doubt the authenticity of his own practice. Instead of fixating on their "tragedy", carrying this personally as a burden, he would change immediate things such as "easing breathlessness and agitation" for dying patients, and explaining things better to "despondent families". This shift to valuing "the circularity of things" breathed new life into Puri, perhaps stemming burnout.

Puri also models Michel Foucault's (1982: 351) advice, that "From the idea that the self is not given to us, I think there is only one practical consequence: we have to create ourselves as a work of art". Meaning is made by 'self-forming' as an art form rather than through instrumental labour such as ascending an occupational hierarchy. Self-forming here is not refining appearance, but rather refining the senses for closer noticing and appreciation of the world. It is not how one 'looks' but how one looks at (or rather, with) the world.

This heart warming tale is of deep importance in the context of this book, where Puri's recovery was facilitated by aesthetics (the meditative making and unmaking of the mandala) and not by functional or instrumental psychological technique. While this is an idiosyncratic tale, it does have wider resonance for medical education. Puri's senses, dulled by the nature of his work, almost certainly clouded by the return of repressed distress, were cleansed by an instant of contemplation of beauty and form linked to a phenomenological insight into the nature of transience. The senses were re-educated through the art of the mandala-making and subsequent sudden (even shocking) undoing – even as contemplative observer rather than participant. This was directly translated into improved patient care as Puri re-framed what his work was about: 'holding' a space for his dying patients in which he did not have to personally bear the burden of tragedy, but rather bear witness to this. Buddhism calls this 'letting go' and insists that this is an embodied sensual experience and not just cognitive. Making the mandala is evidently tactile as well as visual, and the sand surely has a characteristic odour and even a sound as it is poured.

Puri's revelation was deeply personal, idiosyncratic and of the moment. While we need not take it literally as a lesson for medical education (compulsory sand mandalas for all!), we must take it seriously as illustrating the power and beauty of exercising the senses. This book embraces and celebrates *the body-sensual work of medical practice* at a time when sensory work in medicine is described as being in 'crisis' (Maslen 2016).

To be more exact, Sarah Maslen (ibid), from ethnographic studies of how doctors work with the senses, describes a "crisis of legitimacy" in "sensory work of diagnosis" in an age of increasing medico-legal pressures, where 'warm' hands-on diagnostic work is rapidly and literally being taken out of doctors' hands by 'cold' technologies and testing. (Further, there is the threat of litigation accompanying a new climate of acute sensitivity around inappropriate touch.) While technologies are welcome in terms of accuracy of diagnosis, the unintended consequence of their use is to gradually sideline the sense-based practices and traditions of the medical encounter that not only provide an array of diagnostic practices but also afford a medical education nexus for the identity construction of doctors. Maslen is just one of a number of commentators, amongst them physicians such as Martina Kelly, Roger Kneebone and Abraham Verghese, who bemoan the erosion of what is traditionally referred to as hands-on 'bedside medicine'.

But the erosion of hands-on medicine in the face of technologies is not the primary focus of this book, although it provides an important sub-theme. My main concern is that many conventional strands of undergraduate medicine – such as learning anatomy through cadaver dissection, learning communication skills through simulation and learning clinical practice through both subtle and overt ritual humiliation – do not open up the senses but close them down. In contrast, better medical schools do not expose students to such pedagogical flaws, and this should be celebrated. My plea is that all medical schools should critically interrogate and change their methods where this leads to the mis-education of insensibility and insensitivity. Passage through the medical school culture forms students' medical perceptions as sensible refractions.

Refraction

In Section XII of *An Enquiry Concerning Human Understanding*, the Scottish philosopher David Hume (1748) discusses scepticism in relation to the evidence of the senses. Sceptics, notes Hume, argue that our senses are imperfect or fallacious, based on phenomena such as "the crooked appearance of an oar in water". This phenomenon of refraction (light bending) suggests that

> senses alone are not implicitly to be depended on; but that we must correct their evidence by reason, and by considerations, derived from the nature of the medium, the distance of the object, and the disposition of the organ, in order to render them, within their sphere, the proper criteria of truth and falsehood.

In other words, the senses are not independent of the perceived world but affected by that world, and are subject to the exercise of the mind. The senses, for example, can be engaged or disengaged through education. We can take refraction as a metaphor for the education of medical students as they become junior doctors. Like the oar of David Hume, the embodiment of medical students in medical culture, their sense-immersion, offers a refraction through that culture so that they appear in their professional roles as different not only to the layperson as patient but also to themselves. The emerging persona of the doctor must be given 'face' both aesthetically and ethically, so that the doctor can claim 'I look differently', referring to medical expertise, and also ask: 'how do I look?', referring to subjectivity and identity. As a medical education is primarily a socialisation, so the nascent doctor also notices that he or she 'looks different' as she learns to 'look differently' through acquisition of the diagnostic gaze (see Chapter 9 in particular). As senior students and junior doctors, medicine begins to make sense as perceptions are refracted through the increasingly familiar and familial medical culture.

Re-thinking the human sensorium

Here is a patient in a diabetic coma, described by Abraham Verghese (2010): "His breathing was deep, loud, and sighing, like an overworked locomotive. With every exhalation he gave off that sweet emanation – it even had a color: red". This synaesthetic diagnosis should be enough in itself to warn us against a false compartmentalising of the senses. Rather, let's imagine the senses as a dynamic, complex adaptive system with components (senses as 'attractors') working for each other. It is purely for convenience that in subsequent chapters I separate them out. Division into different senses is a rhetorical gesture for ease of understanding.

This chapter discusses philosophical, psychological and biological models that challenge both compartmentalising the five senses and imprisoning them inside the individual. Again, the human sensorium is treated as an ecology, a system, with senses working in tandem. Notions such as 'extended senses' are introduced, relating to 'shared-sense' collaborative work in communities of practice and complex, fast-moving and entangled health care embodying critical exchanges that Yrjö Engeström (2008, 2019) has termed "knotworking" as tying, untying and retying what may otherwise remain as separate threads of activity.

We must go beyond the separation of the traditional 'five senses' to knotwork these, through differing attractors such as kinds of attention and vigilance that organise sense impressions, remembering that there are five identifiable senses alone of touch ('crude' or everyday touch, pressure, cold, heat and pain) beyond proprioception, which is the awareness of one's body in space, and interoception, which is the sensing of the body's interior working; and we must account for the shaping or tuning of the senses by historical and cultural factors.

Finally, we must note a bias to the visual, an 'ocularism', in turn shaped by a dominance of individualistic Western psychology (Jay 1993). Rather, we have a rich tradition of 'intersense' (David Howes 1995, 2003) to draw on. Aristotle talked of an integrative 'common sense', and Heller-Roazen (2007) has extended this to mean the sense that one is alive. Merleau-Ponty (2012), the father of phenomenology, suggests that we focus upon a lived body that does not *have* senses but *is sensible*.

The augmented senses

To limit the senses to oneself as an individual is a category mistake. First, the senses are not what define me – we cannot privatise the senses – but what locate me in, and connect me to, the wider world. The senses are then extended and social. Thus, social learning approaches such as Activity Theory begin with the assumption that learning is 'object oriented' and not subject oriented, where the object shapes the learning and subjectivity (Engeström 2019). Second, the senses are augmented and extended by technologies that are culturally determined. Most obviously, glasses correct my own sense of sight, and the computer and mobile phone heavily augment my senses.

Fredriksen (2002: 71) argues: "The success of modern medicine is closely related to its ability to transcend the human senses". A paradox of the human condition is that we take on trust what our senses tell us, but of course what is perceived directly cannot always be trusted – the most obvious example of this is that vision to the horizon tells us that the earth is flat, and we have no sense also that the earth is moving. A stick appears to bend in water (refraction) when we know that it is straight, as David Hume explores above. Similarly, autopsy findings, imaging and ultrasound reveal what the bare senses may miss or mistake for symptom and cause of symptom. Thus, we must think of the senses now as an augmented and extended system. This situation has been described as raising a conundrum for medical education where medical students become less able to rely on the evidence of their own senses as the augmented senses dominate diagnostic work. But, as this book shows, the education of the 'natural' senses for sensibility and sensitivity affords something beyond cold diagnostic capability – that of warm human contact and development of embodied trust.

Medical education has been dominated for at least half a century by forms of cognitive psychology. This has debrided the senses and it is time we came back to our senses. Medicine is unique in its powerful yoking of abstract science and hands-on sensory practice. Just as medicine deals with the bodies of patients, so medical education should get out of its head and return to the body. This embraces technological extensions to the body that have replaced the fallible human sensorium with reliable instrumentation such as apparatus to measure blood pressure, and dissecting sets and improved microscopes for histological work.

The shift from a first-hand, sense-based experience to precise quantitative measurement mediated by instrumentation is often presented as a shift in pedagogy from direct perceptual experience to mediated analysis. In 1908, the physician and educator Richard Cabot (2018) had formulated a diagnostic method *in the absence of the patient* where "it is easier to concentrate attention upon the processes of memory, comparison, and exclusion, which form the essence of diagnostic reasoning, if the senses are not distracted by the presence of the patient". Thus, *"After the student has learned to open his eyes and see, he must learn to shut them and think*, and when he is thinking the less he has to distract him the better" (italics in original). Here is Cartesianism in full bloom, rejecting an embodied medicine. In this reading, medical students lose an education of the senses and gain analytical prowess. But such reductionism is literally a non-sense – both cognition and embodiment are necessary in medical work as a whole 'body-mind'. Here, the body of medicine has shut down its interoceptive and proprioceptive capacities.

Medical students are not really free to use their senses independently to make clinical judgements because such activities are framed within a socialisation and identity construction process that constitutes a formal medical education. As Stanley Reiser (1993: 268) notes, where the scientific method aims to cancel out differing personal takes on data through repeated, controlled experimentation, so "sensory-derived evidence" obtained from bedside or clinic examinations of patients is suspect in being "sure each person was feeling, hearing or seeing the same phenomenon". This would be compounded if standardised terms were not used to describe the phenomenon in question. Standardisation could, however, be achieved through using common artefacts of measurement and imaging. Of course, what technologies and artefacts strip out is precisely what makes medicine humane – sensitivity that accompanies sensibility.

There is, however, another reading to the narrative presented above that suggests a widening dichotomy between human and extra-human sensing. Here, the human sensorium is extended and amplified by instruments and technologies. We can add to this a social reading, where perception is not an individual use of senses, but rather a distributed perceptual-cognitive activity (and strategy) of more than one person augmented by artefacts. (Indeed we forget that this is already second nature in bedside examinations where many medical students and doctors wear glasses and carry stethoscopes; add to this the wristwatch, bleeper and ubiquitous cell phone with apps such as drug formularies.) As doctors and health care practitioners work in and across teams around patients, drawing on a variety of testing and therapeutic artefacts, so their combined perceptual prowess can be envisaged as an adaptive, dynamic, complex system, or a variety of activity systems generating "boundary crossings" (Kerosuo and Engeström 2003). The senses not only work as an inter-sensory system but also transcend the individual as collaborative inter-sensing.

Reasoning in the senses: abductive judgement

Inductive reasoning involves working forward from evidence to set up a hypothesis. Deductive reasoning involves testing a hypothesis through gathering evidence. There is a third way of knowing – 'abduction' or abductive reasoning, first described by Charles Peirce (1931) as a knowing *in* the senses (Schleifer and Vannatta 2013). Peirce described abductive reasoning as "the operations by which theories ... are given birth", in other words, the embodiment of proto-theory in practical acts. Something is done, and an idea follows that is contained in the arc of the act. Theory is then performative, often muscular and sometimes nervy – in itself an embodied activity. Donald Schön (1990) famously described 'reflection-in-action' as the moment-to-moment adjustment that we make as we are faced with novelty or uncertainty in activity. This is a reflex in the human, who is naturally predictive (Clark 2016). As the blurb to Andy Clark's (ibid) book *Surfing Uncertainty: Prediction, Action, and the Embodied Mind* promises the reader:

> This title brings together work on embodiment, action, and the predictive mind. At the core is the vision of human minds as prediction machines – devices that constantly try to stay one step ahead of the breaking waves of sensory stimulation, by actively predicting the incoming flow.

Such abductive reasoning can also be called 'reflection-*as*-action', where the senses are doing the thinking or knowing; better, a paradoxical prediction-as-reflection, situating the abductive mind in the territory of intuition or thinking on your feet in a fast changing, uncertain context. An activity necessarily has an arc into the future-unknown, the meaning of the activity known only in reflective hindsight. As Florence Nightingale (in McDonald 2009: 723) suggested: "Observation tells us the fact, reflection the meaning of the fact", while abduction collapses these two events into one in which the meaning is already in the observation.

Where inductive and deductive reasoning are the logical elements of scientific thought, Hallyn (1993) argues that hypothesis generation in science can take a third form – as the exercise of a poetic imagination referring to the possible rather than the evident, drawing on the metaphorical. This chimes with 'pattern recognition' or Type 1 reasoning (System 1 or non-analytical) (Norman and Eva 2010). Again, it happens 'in' the senses. It is a vigorous rather than rigorous thinking – more an embodied 'knowing'. Such judgements are also described as intuitive, or a tacit knowing (Polanyi 1983). Increasing levels of pattern recognition mark transitions from novice to expertise, where experts are also wary of premature pattern recognition (guesswork rather than explicating tacit knowledge).

Abraham Verghese (1999: 299) describes abductive reasoning, in this case founded in the sense of smell, on a teaching ward round: "Smells registered in a primitive part of the brain, the ancient limbic system. I liked to think that from there they echoed and led me to think 'typhoid' or 'rheumatic fever' without ever being able to explain why". However, "I taught students to avoid the 'blink-of-an-eye' diagnosis ... the snap judgement. But secretly, I trusted my primitive brain, trusted the animal snout". Norman and Eva (2010) encourage early support of System 1 (pattern recognition) reasoning as long as students are exposed to multiple examples, and this is helped if the resemblance is striking and has concurrent metaphors attached ('raspberry' tongue, 'pear drop' smell, lung 'crackles') (Bleakley 2018).

Verghese's 'snap judgement' in the senses has long been articulated. The philosopher George Santayana called this 'animal faith', elaborated by James Hillman (1972) as a form of reflection, but paradoxically "neither after nor even during the event ... Rather *it is the manner in which an act is carried through*" (italics mine). This is an important insight and moves us on from the 'reflection-in-action' of Donald Schön that suggests a cognitive event rather than an embodied gesture or performative act that Hillman calls 'style', effectively claiming an aesthetic home for pattern recognition. So, a clinical judgement should have form, an arc of sensibility and sensitivity, as well as content. It is a poetic imagination in action. The manner in which the expert clinical judgement is made is what the biologist Adolf Portmann (1967) called 'self-display', an advertising of identity. The paradox of course in medicine is that the celebration of self-display is based on the suffering of patients.

An environmental pattern prepares or educates the senses. This can be readily illustrated in wine appreciation (Brochet and Dubourdieu 2001). A naïve taster simply tastes the wine and may or may not be able to pick out differing smells, textures and tastes. If the taster is prepared however – for example, told that a Californian Viognier is a mix of dry peach with smoky pear and lemon – on drinking, the wine differentiation is easier. In building connoisseurship in medicine, the doctor develops a storehouse of tacit referents as patterns of metaphors, images and narratives, repeated in the linguistic register as aphorisms or maxims (Levine and Bleakley 2012). As an organised tacit knowledge, this again can be called a 'poetic imagination' (Bachelard 1986). Thus, where William Osler says that you must listen to the patient's story because here is the diagnosis, this must be extended to include a pattern of sensory effects. Across pedagogy, such 'advance organisers' allow for bridging or scaffolding between the known and the unknown.

The senses can be thought of as a dynamic system open to development in several ways, and these are amplified in the remainder of this chapter as follows:

1   Affordance (the environment affords or facilitates perception)
2   A dynamic, complex adaptive system (CAS) with the unit of analysis as the individual
3   A CAS with the unit of analysis as the activity or multiple activities
4   A CAS with the focus on the economy of the system (the flow, exchange and vicissitudes of sensibility capital) where perception is socially or ecologically afforded

Affordance and ecological perception: ask not what's inside your head, but what your head's inside of

Orthodoxy in perceptual psychology suggests that an individual actively senses the environment and makes meaning from the sense information – an inside-to-out process. James Gibson's (1950, 1979) 'ecological' and 'affordance' model of perception turns this model on its head to suggest that what the environment 'affords' or facilitates educates the senses – an outside-to-in process, or an embedding and indwelling (Van der Niet 2017). We sense according to what 'captures' and shapes our attention, rather than being passive recipients of sense data. Thus, repeated exposure to patients with similar presenting signs and symptoms 'affords' a perceptual depth in the expert health care practitioner, who more easily recognises such patterns than the novice, because the environment has shaped her perception. Further, the senses operate as a system, not just in tandem, rather as 'intersense'. More, the senses are contained, and prepared, by cultural and historical forms. Finally, where the diagnosis is 'in' the patient's story (an old medical saw), so it is 'in' the patient's self-presentation, as pattern.

Importantly, what is noticed is not necessarily what the perceiver wishes to sense, but rather what the context affords. A doctor may set out to listen to a patient's lungs but, in the moment of presentation, something the patient says, or a colour configuration on the patient's skin, re-shapes the perceptual moment and attention is shifted. Affordance is a matter of what is significant in a total pattern of stimuli in a context shifting through space and time. What this perspective does is to shift attention away from the doctor leading the consultation or examination towards the total context of the relationship with the patient as meaningful. Now, medicine is an act of reciprocity and negotiation within a social context, defined by the future unknown – whatever offers an affordance for the senses. Perception is transaction. Medicine is again eco-logical rather than ego-logical.

If we take Gibson's ideas seriously, then we stop asking 'what do the senses do?' or 'how do the senses work?' for the question: 'what does the environment furnish for the senses?' The functioning of the senses is then reframed as complementarity – no longer 'I see a red rash on the baby's skin' as a precursor to a clinical judgement, but rather 'The baby's skin affords a colour configuration that implicates me'. Is this just awkward or clumsy semantics? Not at all, if you look at the meanings behind the words – the first is a doctor-centred reaction, the second a collaborative, patient-centred transaction. The first separates out the doctor as figure from ground. The second includes all the actors in the scenario as configured and foregrounded. The first is a pattern recognition, the second a patterned interaction.

The main attractor in the dynamic, adaptive, complex system is not the doctor's judgement but the baby's rash (the primary locus of affordance). The baby is the object of the activities of diagnosis and treatment, shaping such activities. From the perspective of James Gibson's affordance model the act of 'sensing' – as 'situatedness' – is then secondary to the flow of embodied information. If we push the metaphor further, the doctor's senses are co-located in her body and in an extended mind that embraces the baby's presence.

Externalism

Externalism (Rowlands 2003) provides a philosophical foundation for the psychological model of affordance and ecological perception that promote 'outside-to-in' thinking. This is alien to medicine's historically conditioned primacy of the individual doctor working as a responsible agent who is also unable to relinquish control (paternalism). Where Existentialism focuses on questions of existence as the authenticity or inauthenticity of individual experience (focused on ontology or being, rather than epistemology or theory), phenomenology focuses upon object orientation or intention. What is it to respond to the presence of the world, or to 'dwell' in it? Externalism sets out to put mind and world back together again, to paraphrase Mark Rowlands (ibid), where Cartesian tradition had separated mind, body and world, privileging mind as the only sure reality.

Adolf Portmann (1897–1982) was a Swiss zoologist who argued against the dominance of functionalism in biology, putting form before function rather than form in the service of function. For example, where animals engage in mating rituals, or display magnificent markings, or set out a territory through song, this is invariably explained instrumentally rather than explored aesthetically. Thus, mating rituals can be read not just as the functional luring of a partner for reproduction of the species, but rather as expressing a large surplus that is the aesthetic nature of the dance itself. For example, birdsong is largely not for territorial marking or mating, but just for the sake of it, in other words, for non-functional aesthetic self-display (Bleakley 2000).

Portmann's work suggests that there is another way to look at the education of the senses in medicine. This involves the double-meaning pun: 'how do I look?' (see Chapter 9). While I sense, I am also sensed, and manage my impressions accordingly, engaging in a set of rituals that are part of my socialisation as a medical student into medical practice. Such rituals, allowing for an exploration of embodied self-display, shape an identity as doctor (or surgeon) and specialist. The senses are then engaged as a system in portrayal of character and in reception of another's portrayal. This serves to maintain socially significant markers such as acting into a role as identification with a specialty, and stereotyping those in other specialties, also making sense of the identity differences between doctors, other health care professionals and patients.

Mindfulness or mindlessness?

If doctors are not wholly 'in' their own minds or senses, but 'in' inter-sensory cultures, how should we conceive of their psychological balance and health?

Mindfulness has become a go-to activity augmenting contemporary medicine, largely as a therapy for the side effects of a highly stressful medical career such as anomie (struggling to find medical culture's moral compass), alienation (no longer fitting in), loss of resilience and consequent stress and depression (often alleviated by alcohol or substance abuse). General practitioners have been advised to prescribe courses of mindfulness for anxious patients in particular, and this is loosely extended to 'social prescribing' such as mindful walking.

While bearing in mind the importance of the Buddhist sand painting to Sunita Puri that opened this chapter, I may be being unnecessarily cynical, but on three scores mindfulness is in some ways a con. First, it can be seen as a watered-down Buddhist meditation technique of focusing attention engineered for a Western 'byte' culture. Second, its epistemology may be reinforcing the very circumstances that cause the conditions it sets out to cure – a heavy focus on self, a movement inward against the world, a reinforcement of personal identity: 'ego' over 'eco'. This, when the primary long-term health problem facing humanity is ecological – the degradation of the environment and global warming; when the world needs collaboration, community, less selfishness and more selflessness and when medicine is just beginning to discover the value of dissipating hubris (Bleakley 2020a). As James Hillman and Michael Ventura (1992) suggest "we've had a hundred years of psychotherapy and the world's getting worse". Third, the point of the Buddhist sand painting – here today, gone tomorrow – was to teach the importance of 'letting go', of transience or impermanence. Mindfulness smacks more of a Western need to 'hang on', to gain or recover, to build spiritual capital out of selfhood.

We need therapies on the environment (pollution, contaminated water, global warming, food degradation, structural inequalities) more than we need therapies on the self. Thus, mortality correlates with both income levels and inequality. A case study would be to switch attention from eating disorders and personality types to food disorders and marketing. Where we are gripped by an epidemic of obesity coupled with a lack of will to exercise, leading to cardiac problems in particular, we need to treat food companies who peddle excessive sugar and additives, and advertising companies who push such products. Mindfulness will not solve this issue that needs coordinated resistance against big business interests. Doctors need to be far more involved in this public health end of their work.

I have argued that medical education must pursue a more considered and vigorous education of sensibility as a basis to developing close noticing. This, in turn, is the basis for developing clinical acumen, especially diagnostic capability. Yet medicine must, paradoxically, pursue a parallel path of de-sensitising – but it radically overplays this aspect of education. At the heart of this paradox, which this book reframes as an opportunity grounded in a contradiction, is the necessity for a parallel education of vigilant and paradoxical attention – and the dynamic between these two seems to me to be the core of Buddhist mindfulness and well worth teaching to medical students as a core clinical capability.

Vigilant and paradoxical attention

Close noticing requires a parallel background witnessing. An experienced and sensitive doctor sits, for an initial consultation, with a patient unfolding a story about a presenting symptom. The patient is placing herself in time and the doctor listens to and holds the story while building up a picture, often from fragments, of a symptom's history. Meanwhile, the doctor is scanning the patient in real time and space, as the patient's body speaks. The doctor notes not only what she says but also the way she says it, the sensory information given off. There may be a focus on a specific issue and possibly a movement towards an initial physical examination; or perhaps the signs are obvious and unmistakeable leading to a quick diagnosis. Or there may be a concealed presentation where a top story is the prelude to a confession – a particularly hoarse cough, sexual misadventures with consequences, drinking too much, abusing drugs, a victim of physical or psychological abuse, been depressed for months now, anxious all the time and so forth. The doctor suspends moralising and allows two forms of attention to exert their powers.

The first, quickly established, is a general background scanning, a free-floating 'paradoxical attention' that does not 'pay attention' but registers nonetheless. Against this ground, a figure is established through close noticing or 'vigilant attention', where the symptom may rest, or call, or hint, or display as configuration, colour, smell, or sound. For example, the doctor listens to the patient's presentation, perhaps also listening to the body in a physical examination, but simultaneously 'listens around' the patient's presenting story and observed symptoms to make sense of the whole – what is unsaid, what strikes the doctor as odd or unreasonable? This is the dance between vigilant and paradoxical attention.

The 'listening around' or paradoxical attention has been characterised by the phenomenologist Edward Casey (2007) as a 'glance'. This has a chief characteristic of an "unfocused meandering", but also a "thickening" in awareness as opposed to the focus and thinning that occurs with vigilant attention. Michel Foucault (1976) makes a distinction between the medical gaze (focused attention as a 'looking into' the body) and the 'glance' that is a kind of 'bouncing off' and 'bouncing around' the patient, an embedding in the patient's presence (Bleakley and Bligh 2009). If the gaze is medicine's mind preceding its body, then the glance is embodied medicine as 'presence'. While Westernised medical students are taught to make eye contact with patients (the gaze), this direct looking is considered rude, even disrespectful, in other cultures, particularly Asian (such as Japan), Middle Eastern (such as Iran), Hispanic and Native American. In such cultures, the glance is preferred (Uono and Hietanen 2015).

Sensibility capital: 'what are you looking at?', or politics meets aesthetics

I have offered a rationale for an inter-sensory model of sense-based medical education and practice grounded in ecological perception, affordance and externalism. This section considers sensory activity in terms of emotional labour and consequent affective capital, generated within a community of practice (medicine) and distributed according to prevalent power structures.

The 'capital' of medicine – folded in to the identity of the medical student, doctor and specialist – is fourfold: (i) knowledge, (ii) activities (skills, and more complex capabilities such as problem solving, diagnosis and intimate examinations), (iii) judgements involving a high degree of emotional content and (iv) communication, including 'teamwork'. Although there is a large cross-disciplinary literature around 'teamwork', this is a term that conceals more than it reveals. Contemporary critics of the loose application of 'team' practices, such as Yrjö Engeström (2008, 2019), note that teamwork tends to be rationalised as effective where it aims for a will-to-stability rather than a will-for-change and the development of high levels of tolerance of ambiguity. Engeström (ibid) has set out a new vocabulary, including 'teeming' and 'knotworking' (described earlier) to better capture fluid, temporary and often improvisational activities needed in contemporary health care, where several teams often work around a single patient over time.

In a case study of teams working around patients who present with atherosclerosis (including general practitioners, vascular surgeons, anaesthetists, nurses, radiologists and laboratory scientists), Annemarie Mol (2002) shows how differing practitioners are invested in idiosyncratic views of the 'patient'. Each practice sector claims differing (and competing) capital in the exercise of care, where overall material, intellectual and emotional resources are limited, and there is a lack of clarity about the distribution of such resources. Importantly, just as we produce capital of goods and services through physical and intellectual labour, so we engage in emotional labour – managing affect or feelings across relationships. Large quantities of emotional labour and subsequent capital are involved in highly charged, intimate communications and examinations, breaking bad news, close teamwork and identification with values in ethically charged or ethically complex contexts that doctors must engage with daily.

As Jacques Rancière (2006) in particular argues, the work of the senses must be regarded in the same way as any labour except that it is affective or emotional. Such labour is productive ('emotional labour' produces affect that binds or separates people) and the capital produced comes to be 'owned' and distributed according to political systems: consensus, existing power structures, hierarchies and forms of resistance or dissensus. Power of course is all about feelings towards, and from, others that lead to judgements, attractions, bonding, intimacies, estrangement, repulsion and even disgust. Medicine is an unusual social structure in that its value system of care advertises lack of discrimination, yet its own social structure is histori-cally hierarchical, masculine and discriminatory, although it is currently in flux. Its lingering inability to democratise (Bleakley 2014) is advertised by the ways in which knowledge, skills and emotional capital are distributed.

Just as patients are not considered capable of dealing with medical knowl-edge, and certainly not skills (despite the availability of information on the internet, patients who are experts in their own conditions, patient support groups and informative media such as television medi-soaps with associ-ated helplines), so medical students are initially bracketed out by experts (senior doctors and surgeons). Capital is retained by seniors and offered under their terms. There are obvious flaws in this conservative apprentice-ship model that aims for a will-to-stability and a processional reproduction of tradition. In the realm of emotional capital – exercised, for example, in communication and collaboration – patients, medical students and junior doctors may have more expertise than senior doctors who have progres-sively become insensible and insensitive through their work. In terms of sensibility and sensitivity, there are tough questions to be asked concern-ing current forms of distribution of emotional labour capital. For example, contemporary empirical studies in general practice education show that the traditional apprenticeship model of passive absorption of junior trainees into a community of practice is outdated, where such juniors act as agents of change, and are adept at re-distributing both knowledge and emotional capital across patient-centred systems (Ahluwalia 2019).

Despite such innovations, due to historical precedent there is a lingering danger that seniors end up holding students' and juniors' sensibility capi-tal without re-distributing ownership back to students and juniors ('I really didn't understand what he was saying, but I didn't dare to ask for clari-fication'; 'I just felt like I was getting told off rather than being taught'). This is akin to a 'policing': 'Move on! There's nothing to see here!' Sensibil-ity capital fails to be redistributed in maintaining hierarchy and authority. Ownership – and then power – remains with the elite. Students and jun-iors of course can resist this, challenging poor teaching styles by asking for greater involvement. When it comes to emotional labour and its associated capital, students and juniors can feel, properly, that they are cheated by a situation in which their own feelings are not valued. For example, a senior might chide a highly empathic approach to a patient by a medical student or junior doctor as too 'fluffy', where in fact it was highly appropriate and commendable.

Five main factors in current medical education frustrate the fair distribu-tion of sensibility capital across experts and novices, such as medical stu-dents or the patients treated by those expert doctors:

1   Experts cannot readily access knowledge and strategies that are tacit in order to explore these with novices. Mechanisms of introspection and reflection themselves have to be learned by experts in order to mine

tacit knowledge and make it explicit. We do, however, have a hundred years of psychoanalytic tradition to draw on to offer a model of how the unconscious can be made conscious.

2   Experts may be reluctant to encourage novices to use pattern recognition in the absence of experience because this may lead to misdiagnoses. However, experts may not judge well how more advanced medical students have already gained pattern recognition ability in some areas of medicine.

3   Medical education still does not offer early and consistent exposure of medical students to patients, relying instead on teaching abstract protocols and logical decision processes such as 'paper' (virtual) case-based differential diagnosis.

4   Students may not have enough exposure to experts disagreeing amongst themselves about more complex judgements. This would expose biases in favour of serial exemplars rather than generalised, collapsed prototypes as the mechanism by which pattern recognition works. Just as better experts read their individual patients as one in a series of exemplars of 'chief complaints', yet still bear these individual patients' 'chief concerns' in mind (Schleifer and Vannatta 2013), so students could be educated through a release and sharing of such sensibility capital.

5   Clinical experts may lack the pedagogical expertise to scaffold learning in novices.

Where sensibility capital is withheld, or equitable sharing is frustrated, in each of the five examples above this produces and reproduces insensibility in novices as an unintended consequence of medical education. The shared or distributed cognition across a group of experts in a specialty is not a handicap to medical educators but a benefit – it shows students how serial exemplars based on real patients (the idiographic), rather than collapsed prototypes based on typical or generalised cases (the nomothetic), inform clinical judgements. As Immanuel Kant suggested, the idiographic typifies a descriptive humanities approach, where the nomothetic is typical of scientific reasoning. If expert judgement in medicine veers towards the idiographic (series of exemplars within a class of symptom), then we should be thinking much more about medicine as an art of judgement readily informed by humanities frameworks.

In distributing sensibility capital, senior doctors are bound by historically formed conventions. A democratic gesture involves sharing capital of sensibility through clinical education, collaborative teamwork, effective knotworking and patient-centred practices. An autocratic gesture involves withholding capital of sensibility from other stakeholders to maintain an authority structure, or distributing capital in ways that demean and mock learners, or restrict understanding and practice. The senses are shaped in particular ways within medicine and this results in a unique type of capital, but the bottom line of human capacity to sense with compassion is part of our common wealth and should be treated as such in medical education. Respect for students' already given human capacities needs to frame subsequent learning of expertise.

The curriculum as a sensory text

Finally, we must also consider a pedagogy of the senses. The curriculum reconceptualisation movement (Pinar 2012) shifts focus away from curriculum content (syllabus) to curriculum process – that is, how does a curriculum 'work' as a system or activity? Curriculum reconceptualisation has two main principles. First, returning to the linguistic root of 'curriculum' as *currere* – literally to 'run the race track' or 'course' – the curriculum is seen as a total event, a complex conversation with oneself and others as a learner in terms of what is being learned and what are its social and environmental consequences. A learner is encouraged to reflect on how she got here, what she is doing and what this may mean for the future, in terms of her active participation in wider democratic society. This gives meaning to her learning experience and, most importantly, allows her to *make sense of her identity or subjectivity*. The curriculum is then not reduced to achieving a set of learning objectives, outcomes or competences, but made porous (and sensuous) by asking how the curriculum is shaping an identity and with what is the learner identifying? In this way, the curriculum is also made responsible. As the patient provides the primary 'other' or mirror for the medical student and doctor so she asks the patient 'how do I look?' for guidance on what to look for (diagnosis) and how she comes across (communication).

William Pinar (2011) describes curriculum reconceptualisation as a four-step process: (i) the regressive: re-telling the story of how I got here; (ii) the progressive: imagining where I will go; (iii) the analytic: what is going on right now with what I am learning, how is it being applied, is it ethical and responsible? and (iv) the synthetic: how will I positively transform the culture of which I am a part? The process of *currere* asks that you become a connoisseur of the educational process that forms you – for example, a doctor as teacher ('doctor' of course is derived from the Latin *docere*: 'to teach'). How will we embed this conceptual story arc in sensory learning? How will medical students not just learn what they need to know and do to practice medicine but also learn how to reflexively critique their culture, re-form their subjectivities and imaginatively progress medicine or innovate?

Curriculum reconceptualisation further asks us to consider the curriculum as a series of texts. A 'text' is one facet of a formalised set of activities requiring the learning of knowledge, skills and values to produce an identity (e.g., as 'doctor') and identification (e.g., with 'medical culture'). These activities are performed, spoken and written. A medicine undergraduate curriculum can be, for example, an instrumental text (what knowledge and skills are needed?); an economic text (what is the cost of training a doctor; what are the costs of drugs within a health service?); a political text (what power issues are at play in medical education?); an ethical text (e.g., issues of confidentiality); a humanistic text (e.g., issues of sensitive relating and communicating) and an aesthetic text (how will a sensibility be educated)? The curriculum as an aesthetic text might also be thought of as a sensory and embodied text: how will the senses be educated to formulate sensibilities or heightened awareness, for example, for clinical judgement and ethical awareness? In other words, how is the curriculum as text enacted?

An instrumental approach to the curriculum as a sensory text would be simply to list each sense and then work out the best ways to educate that sense. However, this is not primarily how the senses work as this chapter argues. Senses might be focused – for example, a current task might be primarily visual such as looking down a microscope. However, senses are usually working in multiples and as a system. As I type this, my sense of touch is fully engaged, but so also is my sense of sight. My hearing is alert as I am expecting a phone call, and I am drinking a cup of tea and eating a cake, so my taste buds are alive and I smell the cake and tea too. But my experience is not atomised in this way. Rather, as noted above, I have the sense that I am alive, in a lived body that is sensible. I am then phenomenologically adept, both embodied and embedded in an ecology that affords a set of perceptual possibilities, some of which I choose, but most of which choose me.

2 'Out, damned spot!'

The abject in medicine, cadaver
dissection and education for
insensibility

Shall we throw physic to the dogs?

In Shakespeare's *Macbeth*, the "doctor of physick" who attends Lady
Macbeth sees the Queen sleepwalking and talking, clearly troubled: "Out,
damn'd spot! out, I say!" (*Macbeth* Act V Scene 1). But the stain, the doctor
knows, is one of conscience, psychological or for 'the soul', despite Macbeth's
insistence that there must be a physical remedy for a bodily symptom, as
"some sweet oblivious antidote". The doctor, however, insists that there is
no medical cure, for Lady Macbeth must cure herself through recognising
the source of her discomfort as guilt; to which Macbeth replies: "Throw
physics to the dogs" (or 'to hell with your medicine'!). A metaphorical leap
then leads Macbeth to muse on how he might cure the ills of his country by
examining its "water" (urine), or purging it of English invaders, using "rhu-
barb" and "senna". But Macbeth's problem is his focus on cure rather than
cause, for his own calculated ambition is the cause of Scotland's problems.

For all its good work (and there is plenty of that), medicine, I argue, is oblivious to its self-generated 'damn'd spots' or stains: first, to the fact that it eats
its young – like Saturn afraid of being usurped (The titan Kronos feared that
he would be overthrown by one of his children and so ate each one at birth.
Rhea the titaness tricked him by giving birth to Zeus and offering Kronos a
stone instead, that he swallowed thinking it was the child. Zeus grew up to
force Kronos to disgorge all the swallowed children by giving him an emetic.);
second, to the level of harm medicine-the-father causes through iatrogenesis
or medical error, largely grounded in poor communication within and across
clinical teams; third, to the unwanted production of insensibility and insensitivity through blunt pedagogy, or misguided medical education; and fourth,
to self-harm: doctors' poor self-care; medical culture-induced anxiety, depression and burnout. Medicine must re-visit 'First, Do No Harm'.

My focus here is on both the intended and unintended production of insensibility through medical education, and it begins in how such an education
can mis-handle the turbulent effect of disgust. I start my inquiry into how the
senses may be best educated through medical education with medical students' traditional 'first patient' – a human cadaver – and the sensory insult

that this may cause: a natural reaction of disgust. It must be noted from the outset that many medical schools worldwide do not use cadaver dissection (hereafter 'CD') to teach anatomy, but it is still, at the time of writing, the dominant mode across North America and Africa (Memon 2018).

Arguments are made by proponents of CD such as Sanjib Ghosh (2015), usually anatomists, that CD experience is essential to a medical education. Ghosh argues, for example, that "shortage of anatomical knowledge could have serious implications on (sic) patient safety", suggesting that "medical schools should shift to dissection as the core method for teaching gross anatomy". The second statement does not follow from the first, as there are many ways to learn anatomy without cadavers (McLachlan et al. 2004). It is one thing to suggest that contemporary medical students do not have enough anatomy knowledge, but it is another to privilege certain pedagogies for learning anatomy.

Ghosh (2015) further claims: "the human dissection room can serve as an ideal ground for cultivating humanistic values among medical students", where "respect, empathy and compassion" can be engendered as the cadaver becomes 'first patient' for first year medical students. Ghosh's claims may be true for some students, but this chapter presents an alternative and more troubling narrative concerning anatomy learning with cadavers, drawing on contemporary and historical sources.

In the UK at the time of writing, 17 out of 37 medical schools offer full dissection (MSAG 2018). Further – a sensitive ethical issue – the sourcing of cadavers globally remains problematic and exhaustive data are not available. In 2012, The International Federation of Associations of Anatomists (IFAA) recommended that only donated bodies should be used for anatomy teaching and research. Habicht and colleagues (Habicht et al. 2018: 1293) obtained information from 71 of 165 countries with medical schools. A summary of their findings paints an unsettling picture:

> In 22 (32%) of the 68 countries that use cadavers for anatomy teaching, body donation is the exclusive source of bodies. However, in most other countries, unclaimed bodies remain the main (n = 18; 26%) or exclusive (n = 21; 31%) source. Some countries import cadavers from abroad, mainly from the United States or India. In one country, bodies of executed persons are given to anatomy departments.

Dealing with disgust

Valerie Curtis (2013: 35) notes how we have, historically, encultured disgust, where we are

> conscious of disgust … have feelings about it … are able to visualize and talk about it … learn from it and about it … make plans to avoid it; and we are able to weave it into our social and cultural fabric.

But, I argue below, disgust in medical education – that necessarily *must* be encultured as it is experienced as a daily part of the job of doctors – is open to mis-management. For example, we do not fully appreciate that feelings of disgust may be repressed and return in a distorted form as symptom, as I detail later. We do not need to wring our hands over this, or worse, wash them compulsively to get out the spot; rather we need to examine our conventions of medical education for the symptoms they may produce, and then make necessary changes.

Where medical error is systemic, individual doctors (apart from a few rogues) do not consciously seek to do anything other than 'first, do no harm'. It is a credit to the 'medicine watchers', such as critical social scientists and educationalists, that they can diagnose the systemic ills of medical culture by examining, like Macbeth, its cultural 'water' to suggest therapeutic pedagogical interventions. It is a tribute to more progressive doctors that they are willing and able to take up curriculum intervention suggestions, such as developing the medical humanities, to pave the way for a medicine of the future that is fit for purpose. And central to this, for medical students, is how they are helped to manage inevitable disgust in the course of their studies.

Disgust is a response to the abject – something that is unwanted, rejected, cast off as terrible, including treating persons themselves as abject (to be excluded from society). In this chapter, I focus primarily not on the subjects of medical education (medical students and doctors), nor on the objects and objectives (patient care and safety), but rather on the abject and its management – or rather, potential mis-management.

Medicine's cloud

The American writer Robert Duncan (2014) in the poem 'After a Long Illness' asks: "what's behind/ seeing, feeling, tasting, smelling"? His answer is enigmatic: "that Cloud!" I take Duncan to mean that his senses were restored to some acuity after the long dullness of the illness that is "that Cloud". Illness can feel like being surrounded by a clammy, impenetrable fog. Depression in particular is often described as a kind of clammy numbing – a 'Darkness Visible' in the writer William Styron's (1992) term, the title of his account of his own melancholia. Illness often seems senseless and sometimes cruel in the way that it strips us of capacity and folds us into an uninvited identity.

Medicine's job is to diagnose and help to cure or manage illness (or 'disease' as medicine prefers). Thus, it is difficult for us to think of medicine itself as showing symptoms or illness – a knot in the timber of medicine that must to some extent be suffered, but is exacerbated by the ways in which medicine is taught and learned. The illness is both a contradiction and a paradox. In a nutshell, medical education promises medical students that it will educate their senses to improve close noticing leading to diagnostic acumen. This is bound with sensitivity – a humanity and sincerity that we have come to call 'patient-centredness' and this extends to democratic engagement with other health professionals such as nurses, as an authentic inter-professionalism.

The reality, however, is that medical education – both intentionally and unintentionally – can be seen to systematically refuse such an education of the senses. Rather, as argued already, I suggest that there is an education of insensibility (and insensitivity) whose symptoms include empathy decline, emotional detachment and insulation, growing cynicism, less than adequate communication abilities and lack of self-care amongst medical students and doctors – all well documented through medical education research (Bleakley 2015; Peterkin and Bleakley 2017). These symptoms can represent an identity crisis, including a failure to identify with medical culture resulting in anomie – a feeling that medicine has lost its moral compass, or does not provide appropriate moral guidance; and alienation – a sense of acute displacement from the culture to which one supposedly belongs. Other feelings can include an existential sense of 'bad faith', where one's actions and values no longer coincide. In short, these various states can be placed under the umbrella of 'abjection' – a feeling of being cast off and cast asunder that disturbs identity, or puts medical education under "that Cloud".

In a book-length treatment of the abject from a psychoanalytic point of view, Julia Kristeva (1982: 2) says: "To each ego its object, to each superego its abject". I take Kristeva to mean that healthy ego adaptation is object oriented: first, I am a social being and recognise that the ego is formed only in relationship to the Other as a realisation and tolerance of difference; and in relationship to the world of 'things' where, as argued in the previous Chapter 1, I am eco-logical before being ego-logical. Thus, and second, the ego is formed within a network of significant objects that define the cultural worlds in which we are immersed. Central to these are technologies that extend our senses. When we switch focus to the superego (conscience, values, moral purposes), this complex is formed in the context of encounters with the abject, or how we respond to what is excluded or cast off in society.

This includes not just that which may disgust us, such as bad food or terrible odours, but also, for those showing extreme prejudice, the cultural 'other' such as immigrant refugees. In Ancient Greece, citizens could be cast out or ostracized, thus losing their citizenry and rights for up to ten years. In a strange twist, ostracism has been common in medicine for so-called 'whistleblowers' (Marshall and Bleakley 2017) who have exposed serious rashes of medical error such as the Bristol (UK) paediatric heart surgery scandal in the 1990s.

A young anaesthetist consultant, Stephen Bolsin, 'blew the whistle' in noticing an unacceptably high death rate for heart operations on babies. Cardiac surgeons at the Bristol Royal Infirmary closed ranks and Bolsin was eventually ostracized and emigrated to work in Australia. However, his whistleblowing led to the 2001 Kennedy Report that made sweeping recommendations about patient safety procedures in hospitals, including quality of teamwork to challenge traditional hierarchical structures to establish democratic inter-professional teams. Disgust is elastic – Bolsin was not just surprised, exasperated and eventually frustrated by his suspicions and then findings, but also disgusted by both his findings and the way he was treated as colleagues closed ranks.

In the presence of what we find disgusting, or what renders us insensible, a values complex is formed. This can go one of two ways – first to intolerance, where we reject the abject in developing a rigid and exclusive values and ethical complex. This describes discrimination and prejudice. A second, more productive, way is to shape a values complex in the face of what we initially find repulsive or disgusting as an acceptance, even cultivation, adapting to this Other as an aesthetic and ethical self-forming. As doctors face ill people, this adaptation describes the formation of medical professionalism. Central to this identity construction as a professional is the paradox that what medical students must do to become fully socialised is to realise that one's old self (prior to medicine) must be cast off as abject in order for a new self to emerge. This abjection by the person of an aspect of his or her self-identity is a small death or an expulsion in which one must realise dejection, and wrestle with the difficult subjectivity position of the 'deject' (Kristeva 1982).

In the circumstance of necessary adaptation to the abject, the superego is strengthened to overcome both ego and id (impulses, emotions) dynamics. This develops a paradox – a degree of impulse control and emotional detachment is necessary to do the job, but this can lead to excessive emotional insulation and inflation of the ego as over-defensive postures (Bleakley 2019). Indeed, this faulty psychological dynamic has come to, historically, represent the norm and even ideal for a medical education. In short, this (over-determined) dynamic can produce insensibility. The extreme example of this inflation is the kind of heart surgery culture Stephen Bolsin faced in Bristol during the 1990s – an ingrained culture of insensibility and insensitivity, a group of surgeons numbed by overconfidence, inflation and arrogance. The subsequent inquiry noted an 'old boy's' culture at work among doctors. This was the 1990s and much has changed in medicine and surgery for the better.

Sensible medicine

To return to the education of sensibility, in 1808, Napoleon's doctor J-N Corvisart noted that he was dedicated to the "medical education of the senses" (in Schwartz 2011: 205) at a time when diagnosis through percussing the body was being thoroughly researched, while the invention of the stethoscope was just around the corner (see Chapters 4 and 5). Over a century later, William Osler (libquotes: https://libquotes.com/william-osler/quote/lbg8c3k) claimed that

> The art of the practice of medicine is to be learned only by experience, 'tis not an inheritance; it cannot be revealed. Learn to see, learn to hear, learn to feel, learn to smell and know that by practice alone can you become expert.

How shall we educate the senses in medicine, and is it the case that "by practice alone" doctors become experts? No expertise is learned just by naked practice. Gaining expertise involves reflection, critique, experimentation and support and exchange within a community of practice – central to which is expert pedagogy. Historically in modern medical education, and still the case in many medical schools, again particularly in North America and Africa (Memon 2018), learning anatomy through CD is the first organised pedagogical experience that medical students undergo and again how the first 'patient' is introduced.

For example, Virginia Commonwealth University School of Medicine has introduced 'cadaver rounds', where, during anatomy learning through dissection the cadaver becomes students' first patient through physical examination, computed tomography scans and pathology samples analysis. Dissection observations are recorded onto a patient chart, and collective observations form the bases for grand rounds presentations. Students then collate observations and evidence to come to conclusions about clinical conditions experienced by the person while alive (Meredith et al. 2019). Here, however, the abject must be faced head-on and hands-on at the sunrise of a doctor's career.

Cadaver dissection

A young English doctor relates how, while studying anatomy through cadaver dissection, she dreamed that she ate the flesh of the corpse she was dissecting (Sinclair 1997). A psychiatrist reports "repeated nightmares about dissections" some 40 years after the experience:

> I am one of those who almost gave up medicine because of the corpses! [...] I still clearly remember this dream. The corpses were after me. I would jump through windows, run, go up the stairs, and they were after me. They wanted to get me. I had this dream many times, I had been deeply shocked.
>
> (In Godeau 2009: unpaginated)

Emmanuelle Godeau (ibid) reports a story concerning "Thomas Platter, a middle-age Dutch medical student who went around France and Europe with his brother during his medical studies" 500 years ago. After "a week of dissection", Platter "wrote in his diary that he had dreamt he had eaten human flesh and had woken up in the middle of the night to vomit".

Here is the return of the repressed – Freud's dictum that repressed, affect-laden psychological matter returns to consciousness in a distorted form. What is denied, put aside, pushed under, ignored, forced into forgetfulness, will come back to agitate, bite, depress, disappoint. In short, the repressed returns as symptom. And so with organisations and cultures, as well as individuals – as medicine represses what it does not wish to face, so this comes to haunt medicine as symptom. Where Immanuel Kant wrote: "out of the crooked timber of humanity, no straight thing was ever made", we can include medicine as part of the "crooked timber of humanity" and suggest that, like all institutions, medicine displays typically unaddressed symptoms. While medicine's job is to cure symptom, both somatic and psychological, it is notoriously poor at addressing its own crooked timber. This work must be left to the 'medicine watchers' – personal-confessional auto-ethnographers such as the American surgeon-writer Richard Selzer, and the doctor and medical anthropologist Simon Sinclair; sociologists such as Barney Glaser and Anselm Strauss; and performance artists such as ORLAN (www.orlan.eu) and Martin O'Brien (O'Brien and MacDiarmid 2018).

Adverse reactions to cadavers – even in medical school – are not unusual. About 5% to 10% of students experience some sort of disturbance to their sleeping or eating habits, according to Mathers (in Bergeron 2005), who for several years conducted a study of how students cope with CD. He said their reactions bore a strong resemblance to post-traumatic stress disorder: "But most of those changes seemed to be temporary ... Typically they adjust and they come to grips and are not burdened or troubled by it on a long term basis" (in ibid). As far back as 1829, the physician NP Comins (quoted in Nicolson 2004) dictated: "Timidity or disgust is unpardonable on the part of the physician when engaged in the discharge of his duty". This stoicism again became institutionalised as 'medical professionalism'.

In conversations with doctors about their experiences of cadaver dissection and dealing with disgust, a few surprised me by saying that they found a kind of perverse pleasure in what others plainly found, at first, disgusting. Jenefer Robinson (2014) notes an "aesthetic disgust" that chimes with these observations, where the abject gives forth a "singular music". Robinson draws on the work of Carolyn Korsmeyer (2011) who describes "savouring disgust". Many artists of course delight in arousing disgust in the viewer, and there is a long tradition, embraced by Romanticism, of interest in the 'sublime' – as, often unpleasant, spectacles that cause astonishment. Such an interest enters popular culture in particular as a species of horror movie, advertising cultural "paradoxes of aversion" (Robinson 2014: 55).

Robinson (2014) argues that fascination with disgust can be read as a source of insight rather than a perverse pleasure, and this seems to explain why medical students both assimilate and accommodate to disgust. After all, in the case of cadaver dissection, it is not death that is disgusting, and not even the preserved cadaver, but the association with putrefaction that the cadaver elicits. Psychoanalytically, in keeping disgust at bay, we might presume that the medical student is doing her job of learning how to master disease. The pleasure is then tied up with keeping-disgust-at-bay-as-mastering-disease-and-contamination: the master trope of medicine. Robinson (ibid: 67) refers to such tactics as "cognitive coping", a rationalisation. This implies, paradoxically, that aestheticising disgust in medicine constitutes a disembodiment – a shift from 'in your face' affect to 'distancing' cognition.

The ritual of CD is a portal that firmly separates the would-be doctor from others. Emmanuelle Godeau (2017), both a medical doctor and a doctor of social anthropology, studied medical students learning anatomy through dissection for her PhD thesis, interviewing 100 medical students and doctors from France, Switzerland, Italy and the USA. Godeau concluded that "the ordeal of dissection" has little value for learning anatomy in comparison with its importance as a rite of passage, where

> Behind the doors of the anatomy lab, the ordeal of dissection separates forever those who will become doctors from those who will not, those who have managed to control their senses from those who did not succeed, those who have overcome the horror of death from those who have not been confronted with it and never will be, at least not as a doctor.

'Controlling the senses' can lead to loss of moral control. In a corpus of 'cadaver stories' collected in the 1980s by the American anthropologist and medical educator Fred Hafferty (1988, 1991), Hafferty recounts transgressions such as male students cutting the penis of one cadaver to put it in another cadaver's vagina, specifically to shock the small cohorts of female students. Today, most North American medical schools still use CD to teach anatomy (although, as noted earlier, globally donorship remains problematic), and recognise it as a rite of passage; but now the donor is honoured, and any student found misbehaving in the anatomy lesson would normally be heavily censured or even automatically expelled from the school. As CD educates students into ethical responsibilities, so it has become part of medical education's repertoire of surveillance and disciplining (Foucault 1991).

Claims that CD is the best way to learn anatomy have been challenged, and there is now evidence of waning support for this totemic pedagogy amongst doctors (Ghazanfar et al. 2018). Plastinated, plastic and virtual models combined with radiological images – and with an emphasis on surface and living anatomy – have, in some medical schools, come to entirely replace CD (MacLachlan et al. 2004; Godeau 2017). In such schools, there is sometimes an option to intercalate for an anatomy degree where CD is an option. Medical students intent on a career in surgery or pathology will of course usually support CD, where it has direct relevance and meaning.

Again, that CD may not be the best way to learn anatomy suggests that dissection has historically afforded "a different role: a rite of passage and creating an *esprit de corps* for the profession" (Godeau 2017). But the rite of passage – a means of socialising into an identity construction (first as 'medical student', then as 'trainee doctor') – does have specific utility, albeit in one sense counterproductive or leading to unintended consequences. Medical students must learn to overcome disgust and repulsion, as, down the line, they will face bodily fluids and excrement, wounds and pus, bad odours and so forth, and, most importantly, dying and death. In order for a medical *subject* to form (a doctor), the *abject* must become one of the central circulating *objects* in medical education (along with cell physiology, imaging equipment, stethoscopes, case studies, communication skills, pharmacology and so forth). The abject is then incorporated rather than excluded.

Again, a medical education is contradictory. Students are taught a specific sharpening of the senses requiring close noticing for achieving the sensibility that is diagnostic acumen (also a connoisseurship). But they are simultaneously dulled as a form of psychological and emotional protection. Coping with sensory insult demands gaining emotional distance. Godeau calls this "the professionalization of the senses" and notes that this is "opened by the paradigmatic experience of dissection".

The first line of defence is physical: lining the nostrils with Vicks VapoRub (an ointment of menthol, eucalyptus oil and camphor), or using a perfumed handkerchief or scarf, is a first step to insensibility as it masks the smell of the formaldehyde that 'fixes' the cadaver. Once, smoking while dissecting was common, as means of disguising the smell of formalin (the aqueous version of formaldehyde). Down the line, however, as medical students learn how to tolerate the abject, defences become psychological and unnoticed because they operate at an unconscious level. As insults to the senses become tolerated and absorbed so the metaphorical skin gets thicker. Ego defence mechanisms of emotional insulation – denial, repression, displacement, projection and sublimation – may kick in, while outwardly bravado and 'professionalism' afford important aspects of 'impression management', where students behave as if they were doctors.

It is the cumulative effect of this repressed psychological affect that matters as, again, this may return in a distorted form further down the line of medical education and practice. First, for many, a kind of professional weariness exhibiting as emotional detachment and insulation; second, for some, as psychological symptoms of stress, anxiety and depression that can lead, for an unfortunate few, to further defence through drug and alcohol abuse, burnout and suicide ideation and third, as longer term character traits such as passive-aggressive behaviour. This adds to the burden of structural problems that beset medicine worldwide – too few bodies doing too much work with chronic lack of resources. Yet, as one might expect, this condition is treated simultaneously as both burden and celebrated badge of honour. These psychological effects may not touch some students, and I suggest that this may not be because they are less sensitive, but possibly the reverse. If CD is treated as an aesthetic experience, for example, this may provide a container for affect that would otherwise be repressed.

Formalin itself offers a literal insult to the senses. Godeau (ibid) notes that

> In the corridors of the lab, I saw a worried male student trying to make a female student smell his neck just after his first dissection. This smell is the first characteristic of the corpse. He or she who breathes it becomes impregnated with it …. Smell is the first evidence of the transformation of the students.

Perceptions, of course, differ. A 2016 first year medical student at Stanford medical school recalls first entering the anatomy lab, where just "A faint odor of formaldehyde hung in the air". However, another student from the same medical school a year later, in 2017, reports that "The smell was unbearable at first. It hit me like a wave when I first entered the cadaver lab and slightly burned the insides of my nostrils". The same student also questioned the value of learning anatomy from cadaver dissection:

> After meticulously searching the cadaver for nerves, arteries, and veins, many of us leave the anatomy lab retaining just a small proportion of what was covered. Rather, most of our anatomy knowledge comes from books, flashcards, and web applications that we study before and after the cadaver labs.
>
> (In Godeau ibid)

Constantine Mavroudis (undated), from experience as a medical student, comments on the "horrific smell and toxicity" of formaldehyde that "repulses, burns the nostrils" and "causes the occasional paraesthesia of the digits even through two pairs of gloves". A 2012 study in a Nigerian medical school involving second year medical students reported that of 75 students answering the survey, "58 (77%) were strongly affected by unpleasant smell of formaldehyde. It was followed by 'runny or congested nose' and 'redness of the eyes'". The study concluded: "Due to the numerous health challenges that formaldehyde causes to students in the gross anatomy dissection laboratories, it cannot be considered as a suitable chemical for embalmment of cadaver for dissection".

Jalles Dantas de Lucena and colleagues (Lucena et al. 2017), in a Brazilian study, interviewed 37 medical students learning anatomy through CD, where

> 26 (70.3%) were affected by the unpleasant and irritating smell of FA, 10 (27%) had no problems, and 1 (2.7%) did not tolerate an irritation produced by FA, not participating in the laboratory practical classes. Exposure to FA was followed by several symptoms: excessive lacrimation (54%), itchy eyes (48.5%), redness of the eyes (40.6%), coryza or congested nose (35.2%) and respiratory distress (29.7%), with persistent symptoms during the permanence in the laboratory for 32.5% of the students.

Noha Selim and colleagues (Selim et al. 2016) in a recent study at Alexandria Faculty of Medicine noted the "Toxic effects of formalin-treated cadaver on medical students, staff members, and workers", where "formaldehyde can be toxic, allergenic and carcinogenic" and that "Evaporation of formaldehyde from formalin-treated cadavers in the anatomy dissection rooms can produce high exposure". In this questionnaire study on 454 medical students, over 90% reported itching and lacrimation in the eyes, necessitating "re-evaluation of the concentration of formalin, proper ventilation and assessment of working practices in the dissecting rooms at the Anatomy department".

A study by Azari and colleagues (Azari et al. 2012) in a medical school in Tehran focused on anatomy school staff members and found a similar profile of symptoms to those suffered by medical students in Selim and colleagues' study above, noting longstanding complaints of coughs, throat irritations and runny noses, burning and itching of nose and irritation to the eyes, leading to a recommendation for better control of the ventilation system in the gross anatomy laboratory.

Formaldehyde vapours are released at differing stages of dissection (Sugata et al. 2016), specifically, as would be expected, after skin incision. Sugata and colleagues (ibid) found that female cadavers release significantly greater levels of formaldehyde than male cadavers, while in their study levels of vapour released exceeded the maximum value outlined in World Health Organization (WHO) guidelines. Exposure to formaldehyde "can cause burning of the eyes, tearing, and general irritation to the upper respiratory passages". Even low levels (0.3–2.7 ppm) have been found to disturb sleep, where higher levels (10–20 ppm) may produce coughing and tightening in the chest, palpitations and a feeling of pressure in the head. Repeated exposure can lead to dermatitis and inflammatory skin reactions on the eyelids, face, neck and arms. Extreme exposure (50–100 ppm and above) can lead to pulmonary oedema, pneumonitis or death.

In a recent Japanese study focused on use of cadavers in surgical training (Hayashi et al. 2016), four preservation methods were compared: fresh-frozen cadaver, formalin, Thiel's and saturated salt solution methods. Formalin preservation – both inexpensive and widely available – was rejected as not only potentially damaging to health but also leading to the cadaver not exhibiting many of the qualities of living organs. Fresh-frozen cadavers best achieve such realism, but this is prohibitively expensive, requiring freezers for storage, as well as cadavers quickly putrefying leading to risks of infection. Thiel's method produces soft and flexible cadavers with natural colours but is also expensive and technically complex, while these cadavers also have a limited exposure time. The saturated salt solution method is, however, simple, low cost and with a low risk of infection, although the method is not well researched.

Naturally, nowadays gross anatomy laboratories take great precautions to minimise formaldehyde exposure, not only in the use of protective clothing such as gloves, aprons and eye and face protection but also in ensuring adequate ventilation. Medical students must also be given guidelines and the opportunity to opt out if they have a strong reaction to formalin exposure – but what of potential emotional or psychological toxicities?

Cadaver dissection and cultural difference

Initial medical education offers a classic example of what Michel Foucault (1988) termed an "anatomo-politics" of the human body, in which not only are the senses of the living disciplined in a variety of contexts, but also the dead are disciplined through medicine and funerals. In Western society in general, Foucault argued, both the individual body (through health care) and the collective public body (through public health) are treated as machines that can be tuned – for example, kept healthy through exercise and diet. Modern medicine has not only treated the body as a machine (Bleakley 2018) but also treats medical students as militaristic-industrial components whose primary purpose is to wage war against disease.

This socialisation into a belligerent medical culture affords a twin identity or subjectivity: as trainee doctor and proto-professional. Such disciplining is unique to medicine where medical pedagogy, as detailed above, has been based on a twin paradox or contradiction. First, medical students must learn to overcome natural disgust in the face of disease and death in order to learn how to diagnose and treat symptoms. Second, learning anatomy has traditionally been grounded in human CD as the central way of overcoming natural disgust against the historical grain of religious and moral conventions. In Western culture, the dead were once disciplined entirely through religious authority. Secular medico-legal authority has now displaced religious frames, with religious ritual as a secondary disciplining.

While human CD can be traced to ancient Greece in the 3rd century BC, Christian creed during the Middle Ages and early modernism prohibited dissection (Ghosh 2015). In the 13th century, Pope Boniface VII banned CD; but the practice gained a foothold in early Renaissance Italy in the 14th century because of some enlightened and influential clerics. By the 15th century, in French medical schools it was common for medical students to learn anatomy through CD. In the late 16th century, Pope Clement VII legitimated the teaching of anatomy through dissection. Still, cadavers were hard to obtain and dissection was only practiced in a limited number of Universities. In the mid-16th century, the Flemish anatomist and physician Andreas Vesalius (1514–64) produced *On the Fabric of the Human Body*, widely acknowledged as the founding text of human anatomy in the West. As well as medical students and doctors, the public, for a fee, commonly attended anatomical dissections in Europe by the 17th century.

The rich medical history literature on the procurement of corpses for teaching anatomy through dissection at modern medical schools has properly stressed ethical issues. However, this has overshadowed important sociological, psychological and anthropological issues. Again, Michel Foucault's (1976) influential *The Birth of the Clinic* argues that the modern 'medical gaze' is a direct product of learning anatomy through dissection. Here, the medical student and junior doctor acquire a unique way of looking at patients, as if at once looking 'into' and 'through' the bodies of patients to make a diagnosis. Such a gaze can objectify patients, reducing them to disease categories. Medicine then provides care and cure to persons on the one hand; but on the other serves to regulate bodies and behaviours, exerting professional power and surveillance over a lay public. Disease categories – particularly in mental health diagnostics – regulate and classify persons. Such disciplinary power operates not just on the living and aged (palliative care and the hospitalisation of the dying) but also on the dead as regulatory 'anatomo-power'.

The above account, however, is culturally biased to Western medicine. David Luesink (2017) describes the relatively recent emergence of anatomy teaching in China since the 1913 anatomy law permitted dissection. The first wave of dissections occurred between 1914 and 1915, leading to a remarkable challenge to previous Chinese conceptions of the body and a subsequent alignment with Western medicine. China has a long history of cultural disapproval of human CD for a variety of religious and philosophical reasons, although occasional dissections of criminals' bodies in particular did take place historically, and a number of historical Chinese medical documents accurately illustrate internal anatomy such as major organs.

However, Chinese medicine evolved without detailed and accurate anatomical knowledge and this differed significantly from the scientific anatomical medicine that arose in the West. From a Western perspective, such Chinese anatomical models, based, for example, on an interplay between abstract principles of 'cold' and 'heat', and 'deficiency' and 'excess', are closer to an abandoned Galenic medicine – based on the interplay of 'humours' – than to modern scientific medicine.

Western medicine has been quick to critique Chinese medicine's non-scientific basis to an understanding of the body. This, however, misses the fact that Chinese medicine places great emphasis upon the qualitative psychological relationship between doctor-healer and patient; and that the Chinese body is best understood as performed rather than anatomised – set within a social context. The individual body is appreciated in relationship to a greater cosmic body, so that the workings of the body become an imaginary that is a reflection of the working of wider natural phenomena. Like Russian dolls, the human body is nested in the body of the people that in turn is nested in the natural world. Each works through a basic set of natural laws such as the interplay between heat and cold. Claus Schnorrenberger (2013: 110) also claims that Western 'alternative' (non-allopathic) medicines have colonised traditional Chinese medicine and misappropriated systems of bodily 'energies' used as a basis for acupuncture in particular:

> The majority of Western acupuncturists adhere to far-fetched assumptions about 'meridians', 'channels', 'points', and 'energy' which have never existed in China. Western acupuncture thus relies on a basic logical error, a so-called Wrong Beginning.
>
> (Proton pseudos πρῶτον ψεῶδος)

Facing disgust: subject, object, abject re-visited

As noted earlier, medicine is a triangulation of subject, object and abject, where the abject is incorporated rather than rejected. Medical educationalists strive to facilitate an identity construction or subjectivity in medical students based on values that inoculate against empathy decline and growing cynicism, treating patients as persons. Still, objectification of patients creeps in, and indeed is justified as a way of protecting students against emotional overload. Accounts of education for such subject positions and socialisation that lead to such objectifications abound, but still the phenomenon persists. Moreover, few medical educationalists explore the territory of the abject – the disgusting and terrible – although, as we have seen above, there are significant medical anthropologists' accounts of medical students' rites of passage.

Most medical students accommodate to the abject so that, as working doctors, what might have disgusted or upset them earlier is now tolerated as the nature of the job. But, as noted, this may be at the expense of objectification of persons: as 'patients', 'bodies' and 'symptoms' – at worse stripped of complexity, character and story. It is, historically, through this objectification (in the face of the abject) that the subject position or identity construction of the medical student as 'trainee doctor' has been achieved. A few students do not accommodate at all and leave their medical training, or do not accommodate well and move away from exposure to bodily events in choosing psychiatry, radiology or laboratory research, for example, as specialties.

The psychologist Jean Piaget famously described the two ways in which cognition and emotional maturity develop – accommodation and assimilation. In accommodation, we move out to environmental phenomena (such as other people) and adapt to their presence. In assimilation, we draw encounters with phenomena into our own worlds or existing cognitive and affective schemata. The development of social cognition depends upon achieving a balance between the two. The development of connoisseurship in sensing – acquiring a sensibility – also depends on gaining a balance between accommodation and assimilation.

I have described above that medical students accommodate to the culture that is socialising them, so that they learn to manage disgust in the face of the abject and come to normalise this, at the expense of objectification of patients. Projected psychological material then shapes such an objectification of patients: but, again, what of introjected or assimilated psychological material? Is this psychologically absorbed without effect or need for discussion? Psychodynamic psychologists and psychoanalysts would suggest not. Assimilated material is potentially absorbed into the psyche through defence mechanisms such as repression and denial, from where, suggested Freud, under the right conditions of stimulus, it will return in a distorted form. For example, as swagger – acting out, inflation, pomposity and cynicism – or as symptom such as nonspecific or free-floating anxiety, depression, anomie, alienation, and more severely, for a few, as burnout and suicide ideation. Actually, this 'few' conceals more than it reveals. If we look at actual suicide rates,

> One doctor commits suicide in the U.S. every day – the highest suicide rate of any profession. And the number of doctor suicides -28 to 40 per 100,000- is more than twice that of the general population …. The rate in the general population is 12.3 per 100,000.
>
> (Anderson 2018)

Anderson points to a domino effect, where untreated mood disorders (anxiety and depression) tumble into alcohol and substance abuse, and then suicide ideation. It is bad enough that we produce this litany of symptoms for junior doctors through excessive work demands with lack of resources in an over-determined culture. It is worse that we might add to this by not articulating, understanding and tracking the education of insensibility through a blunt medical education, again particularly for the relatively, but significantly, few who will suffer emotional and psychological difficulties, even trauma, as junior doctors. It is then even worse that we do not provide adequate emotional support and therapeutic supervision for medical students and junior doctors, or equip them with self-help techniques such as co-counselling (Peterkin and Bleakley 2017).

Of course, for some medical students there are other, positive, routes for psychological re-adjustment after insults to the senses encountered during CD. The late writer JG Ballard (in Boyd 2017) studied medicine at Cambridge University for two years and then dropped out, realising that his calling was to become a creative writer. He had fond memories of dissection as a formative experience, but notes that some fellow students could not cope:

> The cadavers, greenish-yellow with formaldehyde, lay naked on their backs, their skins covered with scars and contusions, and seemed barely human, as if they had just been taken down from a Grünewald Crucifixion. Several students in my group dropped out, unable to cope with the sight of their first dead bodies … I still think that my two years of anatomy were among the most important of my life, and helped to frame a large part of my imagination.

Ballard's writing was obsessive nevertheless, returning over and over to dark themes of dystopia and the abject. Perhaps the essence of his dissection experiences were not repressed, but sublimated into what his commentators have called 'transgressive fiction'.

The physician-writer Danielle Ofri (2013: 6–9) recalls an incident early in her first year as a medical student, assigned to a particular patient, a vagrant:

> Gingerly, I took several steps towards her. As I grew closer, a pungent odor enveloped me, the fetid smell of an unwashed body and moldering

clothes. ... a roach emerged from a fold in her threadbare sweater. ...
I knew that I had to swallow it all back ... This is what I'd signed on
for ... (but) the rancid smell of this patient undid me.

Ofri was unable to engage with her patient and was relieved when the woman
was escorted by a social worker to the shower room.

What a medical student is negotiating here is a complex set of cultural
rules within wider society and within the specific culture of medicine about
what is taboo and polluting to the body. While wider society finds bodily
fluids and waste such as (another's) shit, piss, snot, phlegm, pus, sweat and
blood to various degrees obnoxious, doctors, health care workers and carers must of course pass over a boundary daily to tolerate the abject. But
they do this 'professionally', where their primary role is a sworn eradication
of pathogens causing suffering and disease. This is looking the abject in
the face, where – biologically – the primary abject is actually the disease-
causing pathogen and not its immediate symptom in the form of bodily fluids (Curtis 2014).

Disgust is a biological condition re-shaped by culture. Among the universal facial expressions that Charles Darwin (1972) described in *The Expression of Emotions in Man and Animals* is disgust. Biologists have traditionally
described disgust as the natural way in which we might avoid toxins such
as poisonous plants. Valerie Curtis (2014: 23) suggests rather that disgust
arises in avoiding pathogens or parasites as potential disease: "In general
it's advantageous to stay away from sick individuals of the same species".
Medicine and a variety of health care and caring roles of course demand
that the doctor or health care practitioner does the opposite.

Medicine requires that medical students learn how to quickly enculture
disgust. Curtis (ibid: 35), as noted earlier, says that humans are

> conscious of disgust ... have feelings about it ... are able to visualize and
> talk about it ... learn from it and about it ... make plans to avoid it; and
> we are able to weave it into our social and cultural fabric.

Some even cultivate what others find disgusting (O'Brien and MacDiarmid
2018); and cultural differences cast a large shadow over generalisations
about the biology of disgust.

But, am I making too much of the issue of disgust in medical education?
It is clearly a complex area. Aoife Abbey (2019) dedicates a chapter to 'Disgust' in her confessional auto-ethnography *Seven Signs of Life: Stories
from an Intensive Care doctor.* For her, what initially disgusts, such as pus,
shit, blood, sputum and so forth, again simply becomes everyday through
repeated exposure: "...I probably don't notice any more a lot of what you
might think would disgust me. I have learned in practice to cope with most
smells and sensations" (ibid: 199). She describes coping with "the stench
of inspecting the bedpan of black faeces" to check for signs of melaena

(haemorrhaging from the upper digestive tract into the colon), and "lifting the lid of a sputum pot". But she also lets you know that the trick of coping with this is to "breathe through your mouth" (ibid: 201). This survival trick of course demands education of insensibility – a conscious dulling.

And then comes the inevitable confession: of course some things continue to disgust her that she cannot get used to – "the things that can still really turn my stomach" (ibid: 202). This includes even the thought or image of the snapping and cracking of the sternum under CPR. And: "Even after many years now, there still remains for me something disgusting about ... the smell of formalin" (ibid: 204), returning us to an earlier theme. Indeed, that noxious smell is vividly recalled particularly when she is eating meat.

The opposite can also happen. In the hugely successful TV drama *Killing Eve* – series II opening – Eve is in a morgue staring at a greying, scarred corpse, and suddenly exclaims that she's craving a hamburger. The pathologist knowingly says: "That's the formaldehyde. The smell of the bodies makes you crave meat" (the scriptwriter had perhaps read her JG Ballard). And so we come full circle to the formaldehyde initiation – a stink that permeates not only clothes but also the psyche. Historically, the identity construction of the medical student as 'proto professional' (Hilton and Slotnick 2005) and 'trainee doctor' has centred round the management of this stink.

Let us look more closely at the relationship between disgust (the abject) and medical education (the identity construction of doctors) psychoanalytically. I return to Julia Kristeva (1982: 4), both philosopher and psychoanalyst, who reads disgust culturally rather than biologically, and then introduces an important frame for meaning that again gives disgust elasticity:

> It is thus not lack of cleanliness or health that causes abjection but what disturbs identity, system, order. What does not respect borders, positions, rules. The in-between, the ambiguous, the composite.

This, as Kristeva recognises, is more than an echo of Mary Douglas' (1966: 2) classic *Purity and Danger*, where "dirt is essentially disorder".

Let us imagine that, grounded in contradiction, a medical education must fundamentally wrestle with the "in-between, the ambiguous, the composite". This, of course, raises another contradiction: medical students must learn to tolerate ambiguity at the same time as they are being socialised into a culture that is intolerant of ambiguity. Doctors work every day with "what disturbs identity, system, order" and their methods and means of working engage the "in-between, the ambiguous, the composite". Medical students must then – ideally – be educated into tolerance of ambiguity and this requires an exquisite sense of attention, sensitivity and presence. Medical education's wrestling with the abject might be reduced to a simple maxim through Mary Douglas' equation between dirt and disorder: *medicine is the practice of bringing order to 'dirt'.*

The return of the repressed

As noted, while all health care workers and many carers, including medical students and doctors, get used to the presence of the literal bodily abject as central to their work, let us again return to the dilemma of what happens to the emotionally charged, partly primitive and instinctual response to the abject as it is repressed or denied. Here, we must extend the abject to embrace Douglas' and then Kristeva's suggestions of "what disturbs identity, system, order. What does not respect borders, positions, rules. The in-between, the ambiguous, the composite". And let us remind ourselves of the central finding of the masterful study on the 'authoritarian personality' written in the wake of the Holocaust – that authoritarians show high intolerance of ambiguity, or crave order and control (Levinson et al. 1950).

As noted earlier, psychoanalysis suggests that what is uncomfortable to the ego is reframed through a number of 'defence mechanisms'. The primary defence is 'motivated forgetting' or repression – uncomfortable matter is pushed away, pushed down into the unconscious and left to fester. Actually, what happens to such material – a primary law of psychoanalysis – is that it returns in a distorted manner. The accepted psychoanalytic rule is that more authoritarian and authority-led individuals and organisations will repress uncomfortable matter more strongly than those who pursue democratic habits. The latter are more comfortable with difference and flux.

Other defences include denial, projection and sublimation. Denial may be a prelude or an accompaniment to repression: it simply did not happen and there's no point in talking about it anymore. Or, it didn't happen that way – a denial through distortion. Projection and sublimation offer two other routes for release of uncomfortable emotional states triggered by exposure to the abject. What I find uncomfortable to carry and process in my own psyche I can unload onto another, preferably an already identifiable scapegoat group. For medical students and doctors, this is easy – 'difficult patients', 'uncooperative nurses' and stereotypes of 'specialties other than my own'. Primarily, uncomfortable emotional material is sublimated – the most 'mature' of defence mechanisms.

Sublimation turns raw emotional material into socially acceptable behaviour and constellates around highly socialised patterns of 'letting off steam' such as social drinking, bonding around stereotypes and dark humour (often unsavoury acronyms, jokes, labels and jibes against patient 'types' such as 'heartsink' or 'difficult' patients; but also jibes at other specialties – such as 'dermaholiday'). Sublimation too can shape a personality, typically producing passive aggressive doctors and surgeons who thrive on sarcasm and cynicism, undermining others rather than confronting them. These variously over-socialised (mutual drinking or drug use) and under-socialised (passive aggression) patterns are muted forms of catharsis.

A mature and educationally-stimulating form of catharsis or emotional release would be an affect-centred debriefing after emotionally challenging experiences of dealing with the abject, such as CD, and meeting death and disease clinically. Better medical schools do this. Here, emotional release would be properly facilitated. In parallel, a cathartic opportunity could be afforded by the medical humanities – for example, in drama, visual art or creative writing, not as forms of sublimation but as inventive expression. In line with this, Julia Kristeva (1982: 28) importantly notes that cathar-sis does not negate the abject, but brings it into a "second time", where, to give the experience of abjection expression (e.g., drama), or rhythm and time (poetics) prevents repression of the experience of the abject, giving it voice and meaning. JG Ballard's rich and positive recollections of cadaver dissec-tion begin to make sense as a creative initiatory experience. The medical humanities can then be framed as potential media for bringing the abject into a "second time", a performative and poetic expression. For the doctors Danielle Ofri and Aoife Abbey, mentioned above, medical memoir – also a form of catharsis – becomes a "second time" expression of the abject.

Exposure to the abject in early medical education cannot then be shrugged off simply as a stage of development characterised by 'getting used to it', forming habits, 'hardening up' or taking on the moral responsibilities of 'professionalism'. There is a complex psychological dynamic at work that must be understood and addressed. The vicissitudes of a medical education cry out for psychoanalysis. Not for the sake of it, but to provide a framework for understanding why empathy decline, emotional insulation and growth of cynicism should happen at all. Moreover, the framework allows us to analyse the trade-off between education of sensibility and mis-education of insensibility as a necessary fault line in medical education: one that affords opportunity for further intervention and tuning to allow maximum possi-bility for education of sensibility.

To return to Julia Kristeva's (ibid: 2) mantra "To each ego its object. To each superego its abject", the object of medicine is the patient (appropriate care and safety) while the ego of the medical student and doctor must be attuned to the needs of the patient. This is 'Medical Education 101'. But, medicine has a superego, a wagging finger and an idiosyncratic conscience – a highly controlling, idealistic and aspiring element – 'medicine-as-father' – that has coalesced historically as hubris or psychological inflation (Bleakley 2020a). This, I have argued, is a primary defence against the emotional in-sults of a traditional initiatory medical training centred on learning anat-omy through CD. Medicine and medical education are only now growing out of a century of male-dominated individual heroism that can be charac-terised as a 'dragonslaying' mentality, a finger wagging 'in the name of the father'. There is the lingering fantastic aspiration of dominion over death. The contemporary feminising of medicine is perhaps the most important resistance movement to have emerged within medical education and this is a fast-moving transformation of the traditional patriarchal structures.

From the 'old school' stance, the surgeon Henry Marsh (in Adams 2017) says: "I often think I became a brain surgeon to justify my own sense of self-importance", and "The funny thing about medical hubris is that neme-sis is visited on the patients rather than the surgeon". Well, this is not funny but regrettable. The personality profile of medicine's superego in this his-torical snapshot includes close support and mobilisation of the guiding metaphor of 'medicine as war' (in which the heroic soldiers are doctors). The stereotypically hubristic doctor 'mans up'; doesn't admit to mistakes or failure (cover up!/ ostracize whistleblowers!); is over-determined – for exam-ple, prone to over-testing – through fear of failure; is emotionally insulated (don't be seen to be weak! Don't break down!); sees overwork as a badge of honour (toughen up! Resilience!) and refuses the virtues of democracy and the feminine: a 2016 study of nearly 500 cardiac surgeons working in the top-ranked US institutions notes that only 5% are women (Rosati et al. 2016).

Medical culture has for some time preserved its rituals of signs, symbols and practices that are explicitly anti-psychological. But again times have changed. The new medical education is facing up to medicine's historically acquired symptoms. If, as Ha and Longnecker (2010) suggest, "The emo-tional and physical brutality of medical training ... suppresses empathy, substitutes techniques and procedures for talk, and may even result in de-rision of patients", then we have a moral duty as medical educators to in-tervene. Let's begin with re-imagining how we can best educate the senses.

Doctor as 'deject'

There is one final gloss to my analysis of the importance of management of the abject to the identity constructions of medical students and doctors. Julia Kristeva (1982) discusses the identity of the 'deject' as the outsider who is considered abject and defiled, polluted, and is then rejected. This is the refugee, the homeless, the excluded, the mentally ill and the leper. Giorgo Agamben (1995) has written a masterful body of work on this excluded fig-ure stripped of rights such as citizenship, beginning with outcasts in an-cient Greece. Hospitalised patients – already suffering bodily – can feel like this psychologically and emotionally when stripped of possessions, clothes and familiar surrounds, and then of dignity; objectified so that they feel ashamed and dejected, and sometimes paraded as a curiosity as Jefferson Wong (2020) argues, from the perspective of a concerned fourth year medi-cal student. Here, we can argue that the patient is rendered insensible in the face of the medical profession's insensibility and insensitivity.

Paradoxically, medical students join the dejected in order to treat them. This is the admirable sacrifice demanded by duty. But its paradoxical nature requires careful management of identity. Doctors have, historically, been high status dejects, enjoying entitlements as the profession maintained a high degree of opacity. But this has changed – doctors now seek respect for their capabilities and professionalism rather than status (Lipworth et al. 2013).

Medical students, however, continue to form separate communities on University campuses where the medical school is the jewel in the crown of the institution, and other students perceive them as having higher status. Historically, first year medical students could be easily identified as a closed group because of the shared lingering smell of formaldehyde. Medical students were thus badged or coded by a sense impression as authoritative 'other', reinforced by their own emergent identities as self-inflicted dejects and cultivators of the abject. Medical education has historically located itself in this sticky and ambiguous 'in-between' space of lofty superiority grounded in a desire to get one's hands dirty. Whichever way we look at this history, issues need to be untangled and addressed. Of course this is a deliberately polemical account. I focus on strife because here is where work needs to be done, but fully recognise that a good deal of medical education should be celebrated.

The following chapters will explore the more difficult and demanding issues of medicine's self-imposed symptoms – the most important one being disembodiment – through the lens of the individual senses and suggest how the medical humanities can be employed in medical education to address the compulsory mis-education of insensibility. Let's go to work!

3 How do I smell?

Developing a taste for diagnostic acumen

Two novels, written a century apart, bring the Cinderellas of the senses centre stage, musing on two fictional characters with extraordinarily refined abilities to smell and taste: the first is an aristocrat and the second born into poverty. Both crave isolation from other humans, who generally disgust them. Both also recognise that their extended senses are as much a burden as a gift. Our first fictional (19th-century) anti-hero is Des Esseintes, an aristocrat who acquires connoisseurship through arduous application; the second is Grenouille, born in poverty but naturally gifted an acute sense of smell, becoming the most talented perfumer in 18th-century France, when

> there reigned in the cities a stench barely conceivable to us modern men and women. The streets stank of manure, the courtyards of urine, the stairwells stank of mouldering wood and rat droppings, the kitchens of spoiled cabbage and mutton fat ... People stank of sweat and unwashed clothes ... and from their bodies ... came the stench of rancid cheese and sour milk and tumorous disease.
>
> (Süskind 1986: 3)

Grenouille, the anti-hero in Patrick Süskind's (1986) *Perfume: The Story of a Murderer* notes his gift of smell as one of complete identification with its source: "Grenouille sat on the logs ... He saw nothing, he heard nothing, he felt nothing. He only smelt the aroma of the wood rising up around him ... until he became wood himself" (ibid: 25). In Joris-Karl Huysmans's (1884) novel *Against Nature* (or *Against the Grain*), Duc Jean Floressas Des Esseintes is an aristocratic aesthete who cuts himself off from the natural world (considered raw, crude and unrefined) to cultivate a domestic habitat of sensory experimentation, through opulent interior design and decadent bodily indulgences. Des Esseintes educates his senses through experimentation and reflection in an extreme example, or indeed caricature, of Michel Foucault's (1990) 'aesthetic self-forming'.

Huysmans's novel became a touchstone for the late 19th- and early 20th-century Decadent literary movement promoting an exaggerated education of the senses that modern-day psychiatry might see as perverse – particularly a force-fed hyperosmia or heightened sense of smell embracing the absurdly delicate, such as "dipping slices of toast spread with superlative butter in a cup of tea, an impeccable blend of Si-a-Fayoun, Mo-you-Tann, and Khnasky – yellow teas brought from China into Russia by special caravans" (Huysmans 2003: 57).

Huysmans describes how the aesthete taught himself synaesthesia – the senses working in tandem, such as sounds eliciting colours, recalling the inter-sense argument of Chapter 1. Des Esseintes describes his "mouth organ" – a set of liqueurs whose tastes and smells he knew intimately and whose 'notes' would be combined to bring about a kind of music in the mouth and on the nose: "Des Esseintes would drink a drop here, another there, playing internal symphonies to himself, and providing his palette with sensations analogous to those which music dispenses to the ear" (ibid: 58). Every liqueur was paired with a musical instrument according to the resonance between its taste and smell and the instrument's primary tone: "Dry curaçao, for instance, was like the clarinet with its piercing, velvety tone ... crème de menthe and anisette like the flute, at once sweet and tart, soft and shrill" (ibid). Gin and whisky afforded the blare of cornets and trombones as their aromas lifted the roof of the mouth; kirsch offered a "wild trumpet blast".

A string quartet could be tasted, with brandy as the violin, rum as the viola, a stout or porter as double bass and vespetro as the cello. The correspondences continue tonally, with green Chartreuse as the major key and Benedictine the minor, while a "sweet blackcurrant liqueur ... filled his throat with the warbling song of a nightingale" (ibid: 59). These correspondences are not flights of fancy but based on exactly the same metonymic principle as the 'taste wheel' of wine connoisseurs or oenophiles (see below) where a set of associations provide imagery and provoke memory for deeper thinking. Such correspondences follow an ancient tradition of mnemonic devices developed before books were widely available (Yates 1966).

Huysmans's meditation on synaesthesia through the imagined 'liqueur organ' may have been based on Polycarpe Poncelet's (1755) book *Chemistry of Taste and Odour* first published a century before *Against the Grain*. Poncelet argued that tastes and sounds were based on a common system of 'vibrations' and could be readily combined. To de-mystify 'vibrations' we might think rather of ecological affordances, as described in Chapter 1. Poncelet further described an elegant, simple 'music' of taste composed of seven odours as notes that could be combined in gustatory compositions: sweet, bitter, bittersweet, spicy, sour, acidic and bland. Beginning with the low note of the acidic, each flavour represented a raised half tone, in the sequence: acidic, bland, sweet, bitter, bittersweet (sweet and sour), sour and spicy.

Some humans can sniff out maladies. A retired nurse, Joy Milne, could tell whether or not somebody suffered from Parkinson's disease by smelling his or her T-shirt (Quigley 2017, 2019). Parkinson's is unusually difficult to diagnose in early stages. Joy Milne noticed that her husband was emitting an odd woody, musky odour six years before he was clinically diagnosed. Mixing with other Parkinson's sufferers, she noted that they all emitted the same woody odour as her husband. In a blind test using T-shirts of six people suffering from Parkinson's and six controls, she accurately detected all the Parkinson's sufferers, and also ascribed the disease to one of the supposedly healthy controls. This person was later diagnosed with Parkinson's.

Joy Milne's gift was brought to the attention of researchers at the University of Manchester, and she was given an honorary lectureship there to help with research in identifying the compounds she could smell and to develop a mass spectrometer to imitate what Joy's nose can do. The research has found that higher than usual concentrations of hippuric acid, octadecanal and eicosane occur in the sebum on the skin of persons with Parkinson's. The sebum is the oily secretion on skin found in all people, but in greater quantity in those with Parkinson's, making them prone to developing seborrheic dermatitis (Quigley 2019). At the time of writing, the research has not yet progressed to exploring the anatomical and physiological basis to Joy's nasal gift.

Returning to Huysmans, how might such fantastical accounts or literary fancies be of any help to a medical educator interested in educating the senses in medical students to improve diagnostic acumen? I am not assuming that medical students will share the same talent as the fictional Grenouille or the real Joy Milne, but we can derive some pedagogic mileage from consideration of Huysman's suggestion that the senses can be educated or better cultivated. However, such pedagogic innovation in smell and taste in medical education has certainly been overlooked. The sensory apparatuses of the nose and taste buds cannot be simply worked up like muscles in the gymnasium. Rather, we must look to the techniques of association and the Art of Memory (Yates 1966), where the senses are attuned through linking perception to imagination. This is everyday in learning perfumery and wine tasting and can be adapted for medical education. There is already a working vocabulary.

When Abraham Verghese (1994: 89) notes that "There are so many distinct smells in medicine" such as "the mousy, ammoniacal odor of liver failure", he is linking the perceived smell of the illness to another smell through resemblance ("like"). Liver failure smells like mice and ammonia (once kitchen regulars). One must already have a vocabulary and memory bank of smells and tastes for the resemblance to have impact and then be remembered as a diagnostic prompt. For example, the visual resemblances of 'nutmeg liver' or 'sago spleen' will not work for contemporary students who have never seen a cut nutmeg or a bowl of sago.

The linkage of the real with the imaginary (as memory recognition) is, as noted, readily illustrated through the acquisition of connoisseurship in wine appreciation – the world of the oenophile. While widely mocked for its pretentiousness, wine appreciation nevertheless affords a good model of sophisticated education of the senses. Once you are told to expect the smell and taste of 'dry peach with smoky pear and lemon' (a Californian Viognier), a particularly aromatic wine becomes unmistakeably impressed upon your senses, memory and imagination.

This world – apparently esoteric until experienced – is, again, based on a set of resemblances (the perceived yoked with the imaginary recovered in memory) drawing in colour, taste (and texture) and odour. White, rosé, red and sparkling wines first offer colour associations to fruits and flowers – lemon, grass, pineapple, melon, straw and so forth on the white side; and plums, blackcurrants, strawberries, blueberries, sour cherries and so forth on the red side. The reds then appear more 'chewy' or dense in texture. On the nose, reds may have a tobacco, wood, oak, even 'meaty' bouquet, whereas whites are lighter – coconut, almonds, herbal fragrances, melon, pineapple and so forth. The better the palate and nose, the more sophisticated are the judgements against a more complex range of odours, tastes and textures.

Here are three examples. A red wine is described as

> deep red colour with a tinge of purple. The bouquet is herbal and meaty, with a hint of charcuterie and a rich, soft-tannin palate which is supple and accessible young. It's quite complex. An attractive cabernet with violet and blueberry notes, and appealing balance and texture. There is abundant tannin which is supple, ripe and gives the wine excellent structure.

A rosé is described as a "complex wine with a mix of meringue and lemon flavours. Lovely savouriness and acidity on the palate plus a shadow of oak. Textured, serious and satisfying". Finally, a white wine – "light to mid-straw colour with a tint of rose-gold" – evokes: "nougat and toast aromas plus cashew and almond, with a background coconutty hint of the oak barrel. ... There is some strawberry ... on the aftertaste and back-palate".

Concept maps for wine tasting – 'taste wheels' – combine aromas ('woody') and tastes ('vanilla') (www.pinterest.com/pin/746964288170398993/). More complex charts invoke synaesthesia or 'cross modal association', displaying the colours of the substances creating the aromas. For example, black fruit, red fruit and brown spice aromas are found on differing colour rows. So, the aroma of cinnamon is associated with the colour brown. An oak layer reminiscent of cinnamon spice tasted in a wine is then also associated with brown. Aromas are not recognised 'raw' but by learned associations (famously, in Marcel Proust's *Remembrance of Things Past*, the smell of *petite madeleines* serves to reconnect him to his childhood). (See wine aroma matrix for fruit and floral tastes and smells at http://54waf4aa2j43uxomd3367hpy-wpengine. netdna-ssl.com/wp-content/uploads/2014/03/WA-Trix.jpg.)

A surfeit of the malodorous: cultivating empathy for a stranger's bad breath

So, working with a perfumer and a wine connoisseur could open a door for medical students to appreciate how the senses can be educated for closer noticing. This is a two-part process: the theory offers a matrix between the directly perceived and a set of imaginary correspondences recalled through memory. The practice offers first steps in educating the palette. While only taken up by a limited number of students as an elective special study unit, the Year 4 'How Do I Smell?' module (three weeks of study over a year with a final experiential conference presentation and a written, assessed reflective essay) devised by Dr Robert Marshall, a consultant pathologist, was offered for several years formerly at Peninsula Medical School and latterly at the University of Exeter Medical School. Students work with a perfumer and oenophile and crosscheck correspondences with a clinician. In developing a greater understanding of the relationship between illness, medicine and smell and taste, students often research two particular topics: the history of smell and cross-cultural differences in responses to smell. Both lead to a greater understanding and tolerance for how differing smells may be valued or categorised as unpleasant or disgusting.

However, there is a major glitch in making the transition from perfumery and wine appreciation to medicine: in the former, the tastes and smells are almost wholly pleasant, inviting and enticing. Only when wines are 'corked' do we move into the malodorous. There is learning and connoisseurship to look forward to, with very little in the way of unlearning or inhibition. In medicine, in contrast, the smells and tastes are largely unpleasant or disgusting – a surfeit of the malodorous – and there is much to do in the way of unlearning and inhibition. As already argued, the medical student has to work within a set of contradictions – against the grain or 'against nature' – at once inviting both a ratcheting up of the senses for close noticing and a repression or distancing from the abject and uncomfortable. Medical 'professionalism' could be defined as the learning of the balance between the impulse to develop or sharpen the senses and inhibition in the face of the disgusting (Neill 2020). There must be unlearning of 'natural' disgust in the presence of the abject in parallel with the acquisition of the first levels of diagnostic connoisseurship through close noticing. Again, medical education for clinical work is grounded in a contradiction that must be suffered and cannot be formally resolved. Rather, with the help of the medical humanities, such a contradiction can offer a resource as a central factor in learning to tolerate ambiguity.

As noted in the Introduction, as contemporary medicine relies more and more on 'cold' technologies for testing and diagnostic purposes, so 'warm', hands-on patient contact and associated learning of diagnostic acumen are progressively lost. By and large, diagnostic technologies provide more accurate testing, but hands-on diagnostic work is of course not just about diagnostics. It is primarily about making contact with patients to generate warmth and trust. In such an encounter, we should not forget that the smell of the medical student or doctor is as important as the smell of the patient. We saw in the previous chapter that early years medical students learning anatomy through cadaver dissection may be haunted by the lingering smell of formaldehyde used to preserve the cadaver.

Indeed, the shared smell is part of what has drawn medical students together as a community, marking them off from other student groups – a paradoxical combination of the outcast and the privileged that I characterised, perhaps perversely and certainly paradoxically, as a privileged 'deject'. Despite all attempts to create transparency in contemporary medicine, medical education – due partly to its intensity and clinical work-based focus – continues to create an elite set of undergraduates. Note the rhetoric, for example, of Serena Zhou's (2014) characterisation of the medical student collective:

> We're a unique group of people, chosen from the top of our class from an elite group of students from each college. We're used to achieving and striving to be the best at what we do, whether it's academics, music, sports, art, or drinking. When you put a group of similar high-achieving, neurotic people together, you raise the bar exponentially, as well as individual expectations and competition.

Consequent upon graduation, apprenticeship and registration, the combination of the doctor carrying the suffering of others, the culturally-formed refusal of his or her own suffering and the subsequent high incidence of symptom suffered relative to other professions confirms the label of 'privileged deject'.

To return to the medical nose, there are limits in any case to a medical student or doctor's sense of smell, and symptoms may be out of the range of the human sensorium – then calling for other diagnostic approaches. It has been claimed that sniffer dogs, for example, can be trained to detect diseases such as cancer, where malignant tumours may emit low concentrations of alkanes and aromatic compounds subsequently traced in urine or breath. Such claims, however, have not yet been substantiated by controlled trials, and so remain anecdotal.

Among emerging 'cold' or impersonal diagnostic technologies, an Israeli chemical engineer, Hossam Haick, has developed a proxy device for the human nose (ACS News Service Weekly 2015). Each one of an array of electrodes (made from carbon nanotubes – hollow, cylindrical sheets of carbon atoms and minute particles of gold) has one of 20 different organic films laid over it. In turn, each of these films is sensitive to one of 20 compounds found on the breath of patients covering 17 different illnesses, including bladder cancer, multiple sclerosis, Parkinson's disease, pulmonary hypertension and

Crohn's disease. In studies, the electrical resistance of a film changed in a predictable manner when it reacted to the breath of differing people with differing symptoms. This produced 'electrical fingerprints' that may be used as diagnostic tests. The researchers gathered 2,808 breath samples from 1,404 patients who were suffering from at least one of the diseases above. Success rates were not consistent – for example, the diagnostic procedure distinguished between gastric cancer and bladder cancer samples only 64% of the time, while lung cancer could be distinguished from head and neck cancer 100% of the time. The success rate overall was 86% – good enough to warrant use as a supplementary aid to diagnosis, but suggesting that the prototype should now be refined.

While medicine has long since abandoned the idea that inhaled odours cause disease (e.g., Galen's *The Olfactory Organ* describes how odours might infiltrate and attack the body), medicine catalogues some diseases according to exhaled odours – the smells that patients emit. (Of course, the idea that odours may be noxious remains true in the case of air pollution – now a major cause of death, where over seven million lives are lost through chronic respiratory diseases worldwide thanks to household and ambient air pollution.) Thus, in essence, the putrefying matter of culture thought to be a source of illness (the miasma theory of 'bad air' or 'night air', displaced by germ theory in the mid-19th century onwards) is now located in the putrefying body of the individual patient. This, of course, leads to stigma. A person post-colostomy says:

> I don't think I will ever get used to it. It doesn't hurt anymore – if anything I am starting to feel better for the first time in ages. It just smells. That's the bit I hate: it smells all the time. I can tell that other people don't like it too. Even the nurses pull faces when they change it.
>
> (Freshwater 2003: 45)

Such stigmatising of the sick individual was already prevalent in medieval times. Crispian Neill (2019) quotes from Serlin (2010: 94) that "Skin diseases activated the diagnosticians' senses .... The viscous crusts of favus, for example, smelled to high heaven. Physicians likened the odour to cat urine or mice nests". Aoife Abbey (2019: 212), an intensive care doctor, describes in her memoir or auto-ethnography how she "will not give disgust a foothold" in dealing with patients. A trick she learned is to breathe through the mouth to avoid unpleasant smells, although this is not a good idea when undressing chronic leg ulcers that might stink as unraveling the final layer of bandage "creates a blizzard of tiny white flakes of skin and debris" (ibid: 202). The mark of the dedicated medical student is to learn a professional response to such occasions, suspending the urge to stigmatise. They must learn a technical vocabulary that gives distance from the individual patient but offers the danger of objectification. Shall we say to patients that they smell like cat's piss?

Fruity odours on the breath, for example, signal a diabetic crisis. Foul breath may indicate a respiratory tract infection or undiagnosed sleep apnoea, where breathing stops and starts while sleeping, making the mouth very dry. While tolerable body odour is normal, a strong smell could indicate a skin disorder. A number of internal health problems, such as liver and kidney disease and hyperthyroidism, may lead to symptoms including body odours through excessive sweating. Recognising and treating this is one thing, naming it is another – again, shall we stigmatise?

As an expert diagnostician, Abraham Verghese (1999: 299) "trusted the animal snout" and was able to make "a blink-of-an-eye diagnosis", but he taught medical students to avoid making such intuitive leaps for fear of misdiagnosing based on lack of experience and necessary connoisseurship. Yet Crispian Neill (2019) notes how educating the sense of smell for diagnostic purposes has become less and less important in medical education; indeed already lamented as "a vanishing body of experiential knowledge" by the 1920s, where the anonymous author of 'Smelling Out Disease' suggests that

> The medical profession at the present time pays little attention to the matter, and does not attempt to use the olfactory organs as it should. In this day of laboratory diagnosis, a good many of the older bedside helps have been sidetracked, and among them the use of smelling.
>
> (Anon 1928: 24)

Despite this apparent decline, notes Neill, Andrew Bomback (2006: 327), writing in 'The Physical Exam and the Sense of Smell' in 2006, stresses the continuing relevance of olfaction for clinicians:

> I have come to appreciate one part of the physical exam that cannot be replaced by blood draws and x-rays [...] This part often doesn't make it into my official histories or daily progress notes, but its prognostic implications can be as important as those of the white-cell count or costophrenic angles. I am referring to a patient's smell.

Neill argues that the suppression of disgust in smell and taste in medical education is a matter of 'professionalism', where it is a mark against a medical student to register stinks as offensive in clinical contexts. Besides, as noted, most smells associated with illness are unavoidable and accrue no blame. In other cases, such as poor personal hygiene of patients, reactions of disgust may be unavoidable. Danielle Ofri (2013: 8–9) is one of the few doctors writing auto-ethnographically who candidly faces the issue of doctors dealing with patients who disgust and repel them.

In a story previously referred to, as a first year medical student on an emergency room placement she tells of her encounter with a dishevelled homeless woman who gave off the "fetid smell of an unwashed body", as Ofri spotted a cockroach emerging "from a fold in her threadbare sweater".

So rank was the woman's body odour that Ofri had to force back the feeling to retch. Noticing that this patient, who was in her charge, had not yet noticed the retreating medical student, Ofri hid behind the triage desk "gutlessly pretending to examine paperwork" – dissimulating, managing her temporarily spoiled identity through extemporised camouflage. A volunteer helper or aide – "an older Haitian woman" – picked up the pieces, patiently helping the patient towards a room where she could shower without a sign of repugnance. Ofri expresses unadulterated admiration for this volunteer.

The unfortunate payoff for the professionalism associated with suspense, refusal or suppression of disgust, however, is that positive intimacy between patient and medical student or doctor based on recognition of smell, albeit mainly grounded in offensive smells, is suspended through objectifying the patient. Valerie Curtis (2014) puts another twist into the equation: while "Signs of sickness are some of the things people find most disgusting" – the abject presents literally as mucus, vomit, pus and so forth – disgust, as discussed in Chapter 2, is a basic evolutionary response to what might poison us, so "it simply makes good evolutionary sense that we use our noses to notice illness". Rooting out the illness is, in evolutionary terms, the same as avoiding the potentially poisonous plant or animal.

"There are so many distinct smells in medicine"

A talented and literary-minded young doctor, born in Addis Ababa, Ethiopia, and brought up in India, fulfils his ambition to work in clinical medicine in the USA. Specialising in infectious diseases, Abraham Verghese, Professor for the Theory and Practice of Medicine at Stanford University Medical School, California, worked in the unlikely location of Johnson City, Tennessee with its 90% white population. Tennessee was the last state to join the Confederacy after the Civil War and remains staunchly conservative.

In the very earliest days of the AIDS epidemic in North America, in the 1990s, Verghese, later mockingly describing himself as 'homoignorant', began treating a handful of local people, some of them truck drivers, for symptoms of an unknown illness that later became known as acquired immune deficiency syndrome (AIDS), caused by the human immunodeficiency virus (HIV). Kaposi's sarcoma and pneumocystis pneumonia – conditions relatively common amongst people with HIV – had been treated amongst clusters of young gay men in San Francisco since the early 1980s. But in the relative backwater of Johnson City, Verghese's patients' symptoms were at first a mystery. Recalling that formative period in *My Own Country*, Verghese (www.ralphmag.org/verghese.html) writes of one patient:

> We are nearing Luther Hines's room. I know. I can smell it. There are so many distinct smells in medicine: the mousy, ammoniacal odor of liver failure, an odor always linked to yellow eyes and a swollen belly; the urinelike odor of renal failure; the fetid odor of a lung abscess; the

acetonelike odor of diabetic coma; the rotten-apple odor of gas gangrene; the freshly-baked-bread odor of typhoid fever. But this new smell that is not yet in the textbooks tops them all. Now, the redolence is so strong my nose wrinkles. I ask the students and residents if they smell it? They look at me strangely; one student, an obliging fellow, says, "I *think* I do." It is the smell of unremittent fever in AIDS, fever that has gone on not for days or weeks, but for months. It is the scent of skin that has lost its luster and flakes at the touch, creating a dust storm in the ray of sunshine that straddles the bed. It is a scent of hair that has turned translucent, become sparse and no longer hides the scalp, of hair that is matted by sweat, and molded by a pillow.

Verghese (2010) had already acquired an educated medical sensibility while learning his profession in India, where

> The musty ammoniacal reek of liver failure came with yellow eyes and in the rainy season; the freshly baked bread scent of typhoid fever was year-round and then the eyes were anxious, porcelain white. The sewer breath of lung abscess, the grapelike odor of a Pseudomonas-infected burn, the stale urine scent of kidney failure, the old beer smell of scrofula – the list was huge.

Fast forward to 2005, where Verghese is keynote speaker at a medical humanities conference I organised at my own medical school – Peninsula (Universities of Exeter and Plymouth) in the UK. He is talking about narrative acumen in medicine and how his own interest and expertise in memoir, auto-ethnography and fiction has fed in to his clinical work. He describes the life history of the doctor in terms of a typical 'narrative arc', and how that arc can be disrupted by the unexpected event such as a major illness. Doctors are not supposed to get sick, physically, mentally or emotionally. In the talk, he alludes also to the education of the senses and the vitally important role that the senses play in bedside medicine physical examination and in subsequent diagnostic work. This is Verghese's pet subject; he is passionate about maintaining high standards of the physical examination – hands-on medicine – in an era of rapidly-developing technological imaging facilities such as MRI and CT scans (Verghese et al. 2011).

There are three ways that medical students can learn about illness and smell: read it up in textbooks; wait until it appears clinically and hope that there is an experienced doctor or nurse on hand to explain and explore the symptoms with you and the patient; or set up formal learning experiences such as structured teaching ward rounds with briefing and debriefing, and a special study unit on smell, taste and clinical connoisseurship as described earlier (Dr Robert Marshall's special study unit at Peninsula Medical School and subsequently the University of Exeter medical school is probably unique globally as undergraduate medical humanities provision). The first two options are haphazard. If smell (and associated taste) is important to diagnostic acumen, then formal, planned learning experiences should be available for medical students. But, as this chapter shows, smell and taste go far beyond the education of diagnostic acumen through close noticing. 'Managing' smell and taste are absolutely central to tolerating a medical education and clinical environments. It is one thing to develop a diagnostic palette (fruity smelling breath and urine associated with diabetes, foul breath accompanying pneumonia, the sweet-smelling faeces accompanying cholera, a musty body odour given off with phenylketonuria and so on), it is another to learn survival strategies that block out disgusting odours and tastes encountered daily in medical work and in clinical contexts; to show patients that you care as a medical student or doctor, suspending potential stigmatising and to move through the initial disgust to take pleasure in the value of the diagnosis for the patient.

Inodorate spaces

Students learning their medicine do so with one foot on the accelerator and one on the brake and this has to be appropriately managed. The simultaneous energetics of desire and inhibition, of dual production of sensibility and insensibility, inhabit and are re-doubled by the qualities of the clinical space, beyond the dynamics of doctor–patient and intra-clinical team transactions. Once the doctor visited the patient in the patient's home and so was always at a power disadvantage as a guest; but with the birth of the teaching hospital (Foucault 1976), the patient becomes a guest in the doctor's home (the hospital now the place of hospitality under the ruling of medicine). The identities of both patient and doctor are radically transformed through this spatial shift, where doctors identified as active and paternalistic, while patients identified as passive and regressed.

The very environment students perceive as their primary learning space – the hospital – affords a mixture of odours and strenuous effort to deodorise. Hospitals have an aseptic smell of bleach-based disinfectants (older readers will remember the permeating smell of ether carbolic acid or iodoform – typically referred to as 'the smell of hospitals').

As noted in previous chapters, Michel Foucault (ibid) describes the birth of modern medicine as the legitimising of a power differential between the profession of medicine and the patients it serves through the development of a 'medical gaze'. In this process, patients are stripped of both understanding and ownership of their symptoms through processes of infantilisation, impersonalisation and objectification. Patients become objects within disease classifications, and 'present' as such for teaching purposes, turned from *in vivo* persons to *in vitro* 'cases': from the patient's 'chief concern' to the medicalised 'chief complaint' (Schleifer and Vannatta 2013).

Central to the consolidation of the medical gaze is the development of a space owned by medicine to which the patient is both visitor and specimen – the space of the teaching clinic. The clinic is a sanitised and deodorised white box acting as a background against which the doctor and patient can be starkly foregrounded. The white cube must be 'anosmic' (literally 'smell-less' or odour free) to provide a neutral environment against which the figure of disease is better isolated and configured, further imagined and treated. One must see the disease's contours by seeing 'into' the body of the patient and this involves neutralising the background, including the neutralising of ambient smell in order that the smell of the patient can be more readily configured for diagnostic purposes. The inodorate space then disciplines the patient by presenting him or her in stark relief, open to the doctor's vigilant attention.

Another contradiction emerges – while hygiene is bought at a price, breakdown of hygiene is more costly. Inquiries into the Mid Staffs hospital scandal in the UK showed that deteriorating patient care in an out of control administrative system led to the emergence of malodour:

> They put these pads on the bed to prevent the soiling of the mattress, and like we went in on visiting times, and you walked into the room, you just could not stop in the room. The smell was appalling [...] it became apparent that the smell was coming from one of the foot-operated metal bins that is actually in the room. And the soiled bed pads were just put in there.
>
> (Mid Staffordshire NHS Foundation
> Trust Inquiry et al. 2010: 105)

Tellingly, a further patient testimony recounts an incident in which the failure of appropriate standards of clinical care was directly identified with olfactory experience: "[two nurses] had just come out of the ward and were laughing and saying about the smell in there, and they were talking in general [...] they were actually taking the mickey out of the patients" (ibid: 157).

At this point, we meet three issues problematising the use of smell and taste as diagnostic methods. First, there are physical limits to the human capacity to mobilise and extend these senses, while diagnostic technologies, such as the 'proxy nose' described earlier, may increasingly compensate for this. A conundrum here is that such technologies must not come to displace or drive away the desire for hands-on diagnostic work where the latter necessarily involves patient contact encouraging warmth and empathy. Second, it is hard to judge how influential the pedagogic imagination may be in devising methods to educate the senses for closer noticing informing diagnostic acumen. Educational creativity is required, and both capital for this and uptake of that capital are hit-and-miss across medical schools. It is hard to see a formal, thoroughly rationalised curriculum intervention developing for educating the senses to include rigorous evaluation. And third, the development of acumen in using smell and taste is confounded by ethical and values issues. These include understandable personal reactions of disgust to patients with, for example, avoidable body odour or other personal hygiene issues, at the same time as professionalism demands the suspension of overt disgust in the face of unavoidable effects of illness.

The patients who vomit over you in the emergency room because they are blind drunk will be perceived differently from those who vomit over you on the ward because of illness. Indeed, a host of stigmatising medical slang attaches itself to the first group of patients that would never be applied to the second group, such as GOMER (Get Out of My Emergency Room!) (Fox et al. 2003). The well-documented phenomenon of increasing cynicism in medicine as one moves up through the ranks parallels the phenomenon of forgetting that repression of disgust or sensitivity to the abject was ever a problem.

4 From listening to hearing

The body sings

The 'medical humanities' or 'health humanities' inhabit the house of science. Scientific images and ideas are often intrinsically beautiful, stalking the laboratory, clinic and the imagination of the anatomist, biomedical scientist and clinician like wild animals in full self-display. Such display often presents the paradox of an aesthetically arresting image linked with suffering. In the laboratory, the sense experience can get strange, where science may meet music to realise the uncanny. Yeast, associated with a visually arresting sediment in the bottom of a glass of craft beer, or a pungent and satisfying aroma emanating from a bakery, has had its cellular noises amplified and recorded – an example of 'sonocytology' (Roosth 2009). Where the wall of a yeast cell vibrates 1,000 times per second, this can be picked up by adapted microphone – a scanning probe microscope – and recorded. The result is 'signal' and not 'noise'. The science and the music are bedfellows.

The transition from a cell being spoken for by, say, a microbiologist, and speaking for itself through sonocytology has radical epistemological and ontological implications. As the source of its own 'music' we might say that the cell now has subjectivity or identity, has formed a relationship with its human listener and is aesthetically charged. It is a 'circulating object' in terms of actor-network theory (ANT), where persons, ideas and artefacts are given equal ontological status (Bleakley 2014).

A particularly poignant image to contemplate is the tracking of the rhythms of individual beating heart muscle cells (cardiomyocytes) (Roosth 2009), studied, for example, using chicken heart tissue as the laboratory culture. This would be noise to the human ear if it were not for a meaningful rhythm that turns the sound into a signal. Cancerous cells more quickly metabolise adenosine triphosphate, the nucleotide that stores and transports energy in cells, than normal cells. Although the human cell membrane is relatively flexible, and therefore, it is harder theoretically to pick up vibrations in comparison with, say, the more rigid cell walls of yeast, it is feasible that sonocytology may be a future diagnostic instrument in oncology.

A more pressing issue perhaps than cellular noise is noise pollution in clinical environments, creating stress for patients and clinicians alike. Ambient noise (as opposed to meaningful signal) is multidirectional, pervasive and tolerated only because those who work in it de-sensitise – or are an-aesthetised – to its presence after a while, adding further to the paradox that medical education and practice can educate for insensibility rather than sensibility, or unintentionally numb. For many, the addition of 'background' radio (often in waiting rooms in General Practice surgeries and hospitals) adds to noise rather than signal. Our challenge is how to produce an acoustic milieu for patients, scientists, clinicians and other workers, such as hospital porters, that is generative or blooming with quality and positive affordance. We can address this as a structural problem (common to all 21st-century environments). Ambient noise pollution generally is a health hazard, linked to hypertension, cardiac disease, depression, cognitive impairment and, of course, hearing damage (Basner et al. 2014; Godwin 2018). Excessive noise leads to excess production of cortisol, a stress hormone that damages blood vessels. Symptoms from noise pollution are also linked to social inequalities, where, for example, the less wealthy live on roadsides with busier traffic levels.

While appreciating these wider auditory public health issues, we can better educate medical students in the music of their work, from cellular sound, crackling lungs, heart murmurs, a newborn's first cry, to ambient noise pollution in the hospital. A primary challenge in medical education is to encourage students to read the medical world aesthetically rather than instrumentally. The first rule of aesthetics is 'appreciation before explanation'. Medical students' sense of hearing must be educated and tuned before the functional mind demands insensibility. Ears must be opened psychologically as well as physically.

The body is a flute

The 18th-century German Romantic poet Novalis said: "every illness is a musical problem – its cure a musical solution" (in Horden 2016: 3). For scoffing rationalists, this is a vague utterance from a romantic who clearly hasn't tested his or her hypothesis through a randomised, double blind trial. As a justification for the inclusion of medical humanities in the undergraduate medicine and surgery curriculum, it would not pass muster at hard headed and funding-conscious curriculum planning meetings and boards, probably raising under-the-breath scabrous comment.

This chapter, however, will take Novalis' observation both seriously and literally. If the body is conceived as an instrument, then we are immediately interested in the sounds it produces, normally hidden from plain hearing, such as the heartbeat, breathing and gut sounds. The qualities of those sounds will indicate both health and sign or symptom. The "musical solution" that Novalis refers to is twofold: taking music itself as therapy and cultivating listening to the body as a diagnostic technique – particularly through percussion (tapping) and auscultation (listening). My aim in this chapter is to address the question: how will we educate the sense of hearing so that it becomes a deeper and specific diagnostic 'listening'? My starting point is to note that the two greatest listeners in the history of medicine were also fanatical about music.

Tap some barrels, tap some chests

The Austrian physician Leopold Auenbrugger's (1722–1809) father was an innkeeper, regularly testing the levels of beer and wine in barrels and casks by tapping them. Auenbrugger (2019) had surely drawn on this when he developed percussion as a diagnostic technique, publishing his findings in 1761. (Although the veracity of this story has been questioned by Saul Jarcho (undated).). Auenbrugger described the thorax of a healthy person when tapped as giving back a reverberation that sounded like "the stifled sound of a drum covered with a thick woollen cloth" (Schwartz 2011: 204). He noted that variations from this could indicate symptom. Auenbrugger's technique was based on the fact that in the chest a duller sound ensues when a space with fluid is percussed, where a resonant sound indicates an aerated space. Auenbrugger, referring to the chest cavity, said that empty spaces create the most noise (Jarcho undated).

Auenbrugger's consulting room became a shrine to Echo, the talkative nymph who cannot help but answer back. As Ovid tells us in *Metamorphoses*, Echo tricked Juno and was cursed by the goddess so that Echo could finish a sentence but never begin it. Echo falls in love with Narcissus, spying on him as Narcissus spent hours looking at his own reflection in a pool (where he falls in love with his own image). But Narcissus spurns Echo. Here is a moral tale for doctors who overestimate their own abilities as communicators, particularly as listeners (Ha and Longnecker 2010).

Percussing the body as a diagnostic method and listening for the echo was an imaginative leap forward from the established method of 'immediate' auscultation, used since Hippocrates in the 4th century BC, where the ear was pressed against the patient's body to listen for direct heart, lungs or gut sounds. Hippocrates also used 'succussion', where the patient would be shaken and the doctor would listen for splashing sounds that might indicate fluid in the chest cavity. Percussion combines both hearing and touching. Some doctors will say that percussing a patient on a noisy ward is more about the information given by touch than the sound. In this chapter, however, I concentrate on the sound. Here, we remain in the world of Echo.

Leopold Auenbrugger was passionate about music and his home was a hub of musical activity. He was a friend of the composer Antonio Salieri, who was famously said to have murdered Mozart out of jealousy (almost certainly an urban myth). Auenbrugger wrote the libretto to an opera – 'The Chimney Sweep' – for which Salieri wrote the musical score. The opera was performed several times between 1781 and 1788. Auenbrugger's daughters became accomplished pianists, enough for Joseph Haydn to dedicate a collection of keyboard sonatas to them in 1780.

Auenbrugger likened percussing the body to striking the keys of the recently developed pianoforte (invented in 1700 but first played in public in the 1760s). Piano percussion and body percussion had striking similarities, keys responding to fingertip pressure and wrist torque. But Auenbrugger pushed the comparison further through metaphor and resemblance, applying musical terms to the sounds he was patiently archiving from percussing patients such as 'languishing legatos' and 'yearning diminuendos'.

In 1808, Jean-Nicolas Corvisart, Napoleon's doctor since 1804, revived Auenbrugger's *Inventum Novum* – his groundbreaking text on percussion as a diagnostic art – and expanded it, translating from Latin to French. He was dedicated to the "medical education of the senses" (in Schwartz 2011: 205) drawing medicine away from at-a-distance observation of patients' symptoms to close, intimate physical examination. As we have seen, Michel Foucault (1976) described the 'turn' to modern medicine as characterised by a hunger to "open up a few corpses" through an explosion of interest in anatomy mapped through pathology and pedagogic cadaver dissection; and through 'medical perception' that symbolically penetrated into the layers and cavities of the body, literally augmented by palpation, percussion and auscultation. Just as Freud later invented a 'depth psychology' with its central motif of echoes of childhood, so an earlier modern medicine fixated on the body's depth, its cavernous qualities and diagnostic echoes.

Listening in to the body

One of Jean-Nicolas Corvisart's students was René Laennec. Corvisart became Laennec's mentor. Matthieu-François-Régis Buisson (1776–1804) was studying at the *École de Santé* in Paris when René Laennec (1781–1826) arrived there at age 20, having entered medical school at age 14 in Nantes. Buisson, who also became Laennec's teacher, described an 'active hearing' engaging both mind and ear (auscultation) where a passive hearing was mere 'audition'. Importantly, this kind of 'close' and 'slow' medicine was not simply instrumental but aesthetic – musical, percussive and lyrical. The instrument was again the patient's body, the doctor both musician and conductor.

A mythology has developed around Laennec's discovery of stethoscopy or 'mediate' (mediated) auscultation (as opposed to the 'direct' auscultation that had been practiced for some time, where the ear is placed directly against the body). The established story says that, in 1816, a half-century after Auenbrugger's breakthrough, René Laennec was walking in a park and saw some children playing with a log, tapping one end with a pin and listening at the other. In a Eureka moment, Laennec thought about reproducing this natural phenomenon as a medical apparatus extending and educating the sense of hearing. Laennec said: "if you place your ear against one end of a wood beam the scratch of a pin at the other end is distinctly audible" (in Roguin 2006: 230).

The development of the stethoscope is described in more detail below, but here, my point is to remind the reader of how both percussion and mediate auscultation emerge from the context of the arts – specifically from music, poetry and the genre of lyricism. As modern medicine has progressively been shaped by epic, tragic and black-comic genres (heroism: fighting death and saving patients; the tragedy of the course of disease; relief from the pressures of the job through dark humour at the patient's expense), so a lyrical medicine had been suppressed and was ready to flower: an emotionally-tinged medicine of fine sensibility, delicacy and beauty. This is a medicine of the flute rather than the muffled drum.

Laennec admired lyric poetry and shared Auenbrugger's passion for music, playing the flute, the instrument closest to the human voice. Laennec made many body-musical analogies – comparing the flattened bronchi of the lungs in pleural effusion to the reed of a bassoon or oboe; describing rales as similar to the sound produced by rubbing a bass string and a murmur heard over the carotid artery as a 'slightly diminished major third' (Jarcho undated). Laennec's first wooden 'cylinders' (later 'stethoscopes': from the Greek *stethos* – chest – and *skopein* – to look or investigate) looked like half-size baroque flutes around a foot long and one and a half inches in diameter. Laennec had tested various materials to construct his first 'cylinders', including ivory, but finally settled on deal, a soft wood. Laennec's own description was "a cylinder of wood, perforated in its centre longitudinally, by a bore three lines in diameter, and formed so as to come apart in the middle".

He also called these cylinders 'chest speakers', resonating with the musical idea of a 'chest voice' in singers. Flautists too needed an educated chest action to obtain a tone like the human voice. Laennec's cylinder was then a reverse flute, 'blown' into by the patient as player with the doctor as both audience and conductor – asking the patient to take a breath, hold your breath, cough, breathe regularly, breathe deeply, talk normally. The doctor-as-conductor analogy can be taken further: as the arts of percussion and auscultation took the doctor into the interior space of the patient's body and his own head, so these diagnostic activities are shaped by the acoustics of the spaces in which they occur. A nascent 'medical acoustics' emerges. Auscultation in a small, enclosed space with curtains yields a different result to auscultation in a large, open space, and so medical acoustics embraces context ('stage', 'theatre', 'hall') merging with 'hospital soundscapes' (Rice 2013). Finally, as an asthmatic, Laennec was particularly sensitive to lung sounds. He embodies the longstanding notion of the 'wounded healer'.

So, the aura that created the 'aha!' moment for the invention of the stethoscope was perhaps not mysterious – it was a combination of a psychological and emotional investment in music and lyrical poetry that provided a context for a connoisseurship of the sounds of the human body, grounded in Laennec's own symptoms as an asthmatic and sensitive person, with a cultivated sensibility. In short, a perfect advert for the value of an aesthetic medicine, shaped by the medical humanities. This attitude involved a deep sensitivity to the bodies of his patients, again treating them as he would the flute – 'playing them', imagining the body interior as a set of spaces furnished with soft and hard tissues, organs and bone; vessels through which fluids moved; sacs in which fluids might gather; spaces in which tissue may harden as with carcinomas or stones. This imagination of an architecture of the body is an essential platform for gaining connoisseurship in diagnostic methods.

Hillel Schwartz (2011) notes that where Laennec was tuned to pitch, Auenbrugger and Corvisart were tuned to volume and reverberation. The latter's methods relied on a sense of space and echo or rebound – the 'volume' control. Laennec listened for tones, pitch and vibrancy or dullness – the 'tone' control. The piano is a percussion instrument, the flute one of passage of air variously modulated by stops and openings.

The medical humanities: an archaeological artefact to be excavated and restored

Given a historical background such as the above, it is a paradox that proponents of the medical humanities (and arts), as vital media through which medical education can be enriched, continue to be rebuffed so strongly by sceptics in planning contemporary medical education curricula. Forced into a corner of having to prove the efficacy of medical humanities interventions, medical humanities advocates forget the weight of evidence provided by history. Here, key figures in medicine such as Auenbrugger and Laennec were dedicated to educating the senses and sensibility; were sensitive practitioners and dedicated educationalists with interest and talent in music, poetry and literature; could play instruments, compose and write scintillating prose, their homes open houses for musicians and composers. The proof is in the pudding.

The false opposition of science and arts/humanities has left a terrible legacy. We forget that a great scientist such as Humphry Davy was also an aspiring poet, learning from the Poet Laureate Robert Southey, and from Samuel Taylor Coleridge and William Wordsworth, where, in turn, Davy taught science to these poets (even setting up a home laboratory for Coleridge and Wordsworth). We forget that Mary Shelley was passionate about science of the day, inspired to write *Frankenstein, or, The Modern Prometheus*, through Humphry Davy's discoveries in chemistry. And for Victor Frankenstein, the major issue after creating the monster is: *how will his senses be educated?* For Frankenstein's creation, this would be learning through observation, like a medical education. The 'monster', terribly ugly and ungainly, but furnished with a deep sensitivity, is the abject-turned-deject who cannot attain subjectivity. Indeed, his sensibility is blunted by his attempts to socialise only to be scorned, and this education of insensibility leads to frustration and an anger that is turned back upon his creator. Caliban occupies the same social position in Shakespeare's *The Tempest*.

Read psychoanalytically, we can draw a lesson from Shelley's novel for medical education, re-iterating the argument presented in Chapter 2. Frankenstein's monster (never given a name formally, but referred to variously as 'ogre', 'devil', 'wretch', 'spectre', 'fiend', 'thing', 'demon' and 'creature') can be seen as the return of the repressed abject turning on its creator, just as repressed affect can return as a psychological state such as disillusionment, or as a psychosomatic symptom such as performance anxiety.

Similes or resemblances

Working with the senses is complex – first, the senses are culturally tuned; second, they are part of an ecological affordance system (in medicine, the community of practice into which the medical student is being socialised), which means that the senses are social and collaborative; third, they are highly pliable and so open to 'tuning' into a sensibility or disposition and fourth, they are modulated by the mind and creative imagination.

As with other sense modalities, learning to listen in medicine is facilitated through a vocabulary of metaphors – as similes or resemblances. Galen claimed to be able to discriminate several pulses giving diagnostic clues that were known by metaphors such as 'water-hammer' and 'gazelle-like' (Nutton 1993: 12). We have seen that Laennec in particular drew heavily on metaphor, specifically analogies or resemblances. The wheezing crackle heard in the first stages of peripneumonia was likened to the noise made by raw salt when heated in a pan. The 'death rattle' of mucosal gurgling of pulmonary catarrh was likened to the cooing of a wood pigeon. Whistling from obstructed bronchi reminded Laennec of brusquely pulling apart oiled marble slabs (where would contemporary medical students ever encounter this analogical situation?) – a slick squeal perhaps better recognised as the chirping of a small bird. A patient's breathing with lung disease produced, for Laennec, a sound like "a fly buzzing in a porcelain vase", and a tinkling similar to that of a small bell just as it stops ringing. Heart symptoms would be recognised as like a rasp or saw, or the "sighing of the wind through a keyhole". (Today a familiar metaphor in lung auscultation is to hear 'crackles' that resemble the rustling of cellophane, or the undoing of Velcro.)

For Laennec in particular, resemblances abounded and, unfortunately, the vocabulary of auscultation became overly complex and inflated. Students are overwhelmed rather than helped when this vocabulary becomes too elaborate and connoisseurship seems to be preserved for the very few. Indeed, as Saul Jarcho (undated) notes, if even an experienced clinician today repeats the first technique that Auenbrugger devised for percussion, and the rolled up quire of paper that inspired Laennec to develop the stethoscope, it is very difficult to pick up the specific sonic information that these groundbreaking clinicians described. Jarcho does not doubt their honesty in reporting, suggesting that their senses of hearing, as musicians, were exceptional, certainly extremely finely attuned.

Historical changes of the kind so far outlined are accompanied by cultural differences. That auscultation is shaped culturally can be illustrated by comparing a European and Indian subcontinent response to putting the stethoscope to a patient's chest. A European doctor, educated in a Shakespearean climate of language soaked up since schooldays, might hear the normal heartbeat in terms of iambic pentameter rhythm: lub-dup/lub-dup/lub-dup/lub-dup, where a South Indian doctor might hear the heartbeat in terms of Carnatic beats: tak-dina-din. (Imagine this as played on a tabla.) This can be extended to rhythmic sounds from the digestive system and the lung that could be registered either in European musical and poetic diction, or in Carnatic beats. What the clinician is tuned to are variations from standard beats in either format, indicating, for example, tumours in the lungs, leaking heart valves or heart muscle problems. Dr S. Elango, once vice-president of the Indian Public Health Association, produced a Compact Disc of Carnatic beats with the claim:

> While it takes years of experience for a specialist to realise that something is wrong with your heart by listening to its beat, this CD of Carnatic beats, corresponding to different abnormal organ rhythms, will help medical students learn and remember the sounds in a short time. This will help them pick up diseases early and also ask for the right tests.
> (Site now unavailable)

Supplementing such an acute auditory capability is an imagination of space, a body-architectural imagination, mentioned earlier. Contemporary reports mention Laennec's diagnosis of a 'vast tuberculous excavation' (tuberculosis) occupying the entire superior lobe of the right lung that was confirmed at post-mortem examination. Sounds were imagined as emanating from restricted spaces, or, conversely, filling an auditorium: body cavities expanded to 'vast' caverns; the space 'excavated' by the intruding 'liquid, yellow, puriform matter' found at post-mortem. Laennec mapped a medical geography through sound in which the inner body is the landscape: Echo redux.

Listening for evidence

Auscultation examination of a female patient for a doctor in the early 1800s, especially of the chest (for heart or lung symptoms), was a sensitive issue due to invasion of privacy or perceived inappropriate touch, despite professional demeanour. Michel Foucault (1976) in *The Birth of the Clinic* claimed that one of the most important cultural shifts in medicine was the move from home visits to the establishment of teaching hospitals, where patients were the visitors. In the home, especially amongst the wealthy or privileged, the doctor is guest and the patient host, and the doctor's range of physical examination possibilities are restricted by this power relationship within a code of manners. Where the patient visited the clinic, the doctor was now host and could exert a greater amount of control over the situation. The power relationship between doctor and patient was now reversed. However, a code of manners still prevailed that in particular restricted the male doctor's freedom to perform necessary intimate examinations on women. The introduction of the stethoscope gave doctors an opportunity to literally distance themselves not only from genteel women who may be upset by even professional intimacy but, on the other side of the coin, from "the unwashed poor of the hospital or dispensary" where the stethoscope provided "protection ... to his (the doctor's) sensibilities" (Nicolson 2004: 152–53).

Again, here is the mediate auscultation Creation Myth: faced with a young but overweight woman patient, in 1816, René Laennac – working at the *Necker-Enfants Malades* hospital in Paris – improvised by tightly rolling up a quire of notepaper to make a long funnel shaped tube. He was astounded by the amplification gained of heart and lung sounds. He progressed the crude paper stethoscope – from the Greek *stethos* (chest) and *scopos* (examination) – into a sturdy wooden tube, as noted earlier. Although monaural, awkward to use and slightly abrasive on the patient's skin, the stethoscope revolutionised listening in medicine. Despite some early advocates, it took a decade for the stethoscope to be established as a common diagnostic tool in UK teaching hospitals such as Edinburgh and London (ibid), where a combination of stubborn prejudice from older doctors, and slow learning because of lack of teachers, prevailed against a background of suspicion of anything of French origin (the Napoleonic Wars had only finished in 1815).

Pierre Adolphe Piorry reduced the diameter of the stethoscope from one and a half inches to the width of a finger in 1828, and introduced a cone-shaped chest piece that tapered into a thinner earpiece. The latter allowed for a better seal at the ear. A British doctor, Golding Bird, further advanced stethoscope design by introducing a flexible tube in 1840. In 1843, Charles James Blasius Williams designed a binaural stethoscope with a cone-shaped chest piece attaching to a connection with two bent lead pipes. This design was refined in 1851 by the Irish physician Arthur Leared and in 1852 by George Camman in New York. Camman also wrote an influential work on diagnosis by auscultation as a consequence of refining the instrument. By 1855, he had developed a model with flexible woven tubing, a wooden chest piece, ivory earpieces and a rubber band to hold the stethoscope in place on the doctor's head. Camman developed his design for commercial production but did not patent it as he believed the stethoscope should be freely available to every doctor.

Camman's stethoscope was relatively complex and stiff. The ivory earpieces were connected to metal tubes that were further connected to two tubes covered in wound silk. These joined a common, hollow ball that amplified the sound from the chest piece – a conical shaped bell. Later tube design improved flexibility – a stethoscope with a tube made from the tough plastic substance gutta-percha was displayed at the Great Exhibition in London as early as 1851. By the 1890s, the flexible plastic stethoscope with two earpieces and a bell-like end was the norm. Use of the stethoscope advanced beyond the chest cavity to bowel sounds and listening to the developing foetus. By the 1940s, a stethoscope had been designed with two sides, one for the cardiovascular system and one for the respiratory system. By the 1970s, electronic stethoscopes had been introduced that amplify sound and produced graphs shifting sense dominance from hearing back to the culturally favoured looking. Stethoscopes had become lighter, more flexible and acoustically sophisticated as they filtered out external noise.

As the stethoscope was developed, with a flexible rather than a rigid tube, this allowed the doctor to come face to face with the patient again. A narrative could be taken simultaneously from the patient's conscious and deliberated story and the unfiltered, unconscious voices of the inner body. As stethoscopes became integral to medicine, they also became its leading symbol. Medical students developing identities as doctors wore white coats and sported stethoscopes – often given to them during induction into medical school as an initiation ritual.

Just as the stethoscope was once a technology that significantly enhanced listening, so new technologies have eclipsed the stethoscope and the power of auscultation as a diagnostic device. The stethoscope has become more a symbol of the profession rather than a necessary tool (English 2016). The availability of a variety of coloured stethoscopes allowed students to personalise an otherwise universal symbol. Future generations of students will have less and less need for bedside diagnostic skills of auscultation, percussion and palpation as technologies and tests replace these. In an era of political correctness and high standards of professionalism, touch is increasingly taboo even in medicine, except for necessary clinical investigations. Yet bedside diagnostic talk and touch, listening and sensitive examination or appropriate touch for reassurance and empathy are important for successful clinical encounters (Kelly et al. 2014), as repeated insistently in this book.

Ditch the stethoscope?

The doctor's famous white coat (in North America worn short in medical students and long in qualified doctors) is not a diagnostic device, but it may act as a health intervention, comforting patients that they are, supposedly, in the hands of an expert or at least will be steered towards expertise. But white coats are actually a health hazard, gathering and harbouring bugs that could lead to hospital-acquired infections for vulnerable patients. The UK National Health Service properly ditched the wearing of white coats (along with ties) for medical students and doctors some time ago. North America and other regions stubbornly hang on to the white coat, even making the acquisition of one's first white coat and stethoscope an initiation ritual. Just as the white coat is purely symbolic, will the stethoscope go the same way?

We can amplify, digitise, filter and record sounds from the heart, lungs, bowels and blood vessels, and have a stethoscope that can reproduce these sounds – indicating symptoms – on a mobile phone app and send them directly to an electronic patient record (Bernstein 2016). Further, we have pocket-sized ultrasound equipment and sophisticated echocardiograms, and there are algorithms that can analyse the data to offer a differential diagnosis.

Sanjiv Kaul (2014), in an editorial for *Echo Research and Practice*, says: "It is time to discard the inaccurate albeit iconic stethoscope and join the rest of mankind in the technology revolution!" He suggests that technologies such as pocket ultrasound devices will inevitably supplant the stethoscope for cardiac investigations. But also, while medical students and junior doctors consistently remain poor at identifying cardiac abnormalities – typically recognising less than 40% of heart sounds heard through cardiac auscultation – and where simulation training does not help (Finley 2011), let's face the music and adapt. Similar calls have been made since at least the beginning of the new millennium. Fredriksen (2002), however, says: "the stethoscope is not obsolete. It is still a central part of medical practice".

Mangione and Nieman (1997) noted that cardiac auscultatory skills of junior doctors were "disturbingly" poor, suggesting that either better teaching methods must be found, or new technologies employed. Studies a decade later (e.g., Vukanovic-Criley et al. 2006) noted exactly the same deficiencies, and again calls were made for better teaching methods and more widespread use of new technologies combining audio with visual information. Such methods had been tried in medical education – for example, Woywodt and colleagues (2004) linked an electronic stethoscope to a laptop, using software to create a visualisation and amplification of auscultatory findings – but retention of skills remained poor.

In 2012, Mount Sinai School of Medicine in New York began giving medical students handheld ultrasound devices that can generate real-time images of the heart at the bedside, switching of course from 'listening' to 'looking', in line with Western culture's preferred perceptual mode (ocularcentrism). The rationale was that auscultation is superfluous for heart sounds, although still useful for lung and bowel sounds (see Marwick et al. 2014). Clinicians wary of the widespread displacement of the stethoscope again say that this is part of a disturbing wider movement in modern medicine sceptical of hands-on physical examinations where laboratory testing offers a far more accurate diagnostic tool. However, like 'overdiagnosis' (Welch et al. 2011), 'overtesting' is seen as a symptom of modern medicine's anxiety over misdiagnoses and subsequent potential patient litigation, although such overtesting can put a strain on health system resources.

Asghar and colleagues (Asghar et al. 2010: 283) reported a decade ago that approximately three-quarters of American interns and two-thirds of cardiology trainees "no longer receive formal teaching in cardiac auscultation". The authors bemoan this situation where traditional bedside physical examination "can avoid the potential of 'over-investigating' patients and causing unnecessary anxiety". They suggest mixing and matching bedside learning with (i) computer-based teaching, (ii) use of interactive CD-ROMs, (iii) virtual patient examination, (iv) use of web-based resources (such as MurmurLab.org and MurmurQuz.org) and (v) intensive master class approaches working with a master auscultator. Binka et al. (2016) suggest that the "solution is simple" to the longstanding issue of poor performance on cardiac auscultation – it's the Carnegie Hall joke: 'Musician: "excuse me, how do I get to Carnegie Hall?" Bystander: "Practice, practice, practice!"' These authors suggest "intensive repetition listening at least 400 times to each heart sound". Indeed, their study of an experimental and control group's performance does show significant increase in those who adopted the repetitive listening practice. What they did not show was whether or not such effects decayed over time without top-up practice.

But this is a purely instrumental view of skills learning, echoing the infamous '10,000 hours rule' of expertise introduced by Malcolm Gladwell (2008) – or 'practice, practice, practice!' First, after 10,000 hours, why do some people flat line, or show only baseline expertise (competence), where others show connoisseurship and expanding potential (capability)? Second, while individual practice is inevitable, the nature of skills learning is often based in a community of practice, where collaborative and 'distributed' expertise offer different models to individual expertise and shared load and techniques can radically reduce needed practice time (Engeström 2019). Again, does an individual doctor need to possess a set of skills at a level of expertise that is outplayed by technologies (distributed learning) and can be shared across a team working around a patient? To his credit, Gladwell himself says that practice is not the only factor in gaining expertise. There are, for example, natural differences in dexterity.

We have seen how bedside physical examination expertise shapes both the therapeutic relationship with a patient and the doctor's identity. Such an education of the senses leads to both a sensibility – an aesthetic and ethics of practice – and a sensitivity, the forming of a therapeutic relationship with patients. Both involve intensive affective colouration, realised in the management of the return of repressed emotions from a medical education such as the shock of contact with death and disgust, and the transference relationship with patients and colleagues. The latter opens the door to power relationships, adding a political dimension to the aesthetic and ethical issues already mentioned.

Medicine becomes a practice of qualities as well as quantities, challenging instrumentalism or functionalism. Instrumental practice is embedded in a complex of factors including the varying quality of the communities of practice in which skills such auscultation are acquired, the emotional investment in each act of practice and the quality of relationship between the doctor and the patient. Again, hands-on capabilities such as percussion and auscultation have a wider arc of reference than the purely functional. In this role, such capabilities are still central to diagnostic acumen, because they elicit more than bodily signs – they stimulate conversation about those signs, giving depth, texture and meaning to the patient's narrative.

However, we cannot throw out the baby with the bathwater as far as a repertoire of physical examination skills is concerned. A champion of such a repertoire, as noted in previous chapters, is Abraham Verghese. He has developed an educational programme in physical examination skills at Stanford University Medical School – 'Stanford Medicine 25' (https://stanfordmedicine25.stanford.edu) – which teaches 25 basic examination techniques including percussion, palpation and auscultation techniques. Verghese is a tireless champion of the physical examination done well. Like Auenbrugger and Laennec who were musicians, composers and connoisseurs of sound, Verghese is a highly accomplished writer, of auto-ethnography, memoir and fiction. This sensibility feeds into his medicine as his medicine feeds back into literary representations, again illustrating the medical humanities at work in the wild.

5 Medical students learn 'sonic alignment'

The medical humanities and listening

Ambient and elective noise in clinical spaces

'Live from the Operating Room' is a CD of classical piano music by Dr Jorge Camara, a renowned North American ophthalmologist and classically trained pianist (www.livefromtheor.com/themusic.html). The music was recorded in the operating theatre of what was St Francis Medical Center in Honolulu, now Hawaii Medical Center East. Camara reportedly played for 115 of his patients, aged 49–79, before their first eye operations. In the *Medscape Journal of Medicine* (Camara et al. 2008), Camara and colleagues claimed that listening to the music prior to operations had "profound" effects upon the patients' physiology, significantly lowering blood pressure, heart and respiratory rates prior to sedation or pain medication.

In my experience of researching teamwork in operating theatres over many years, nobody is more sceptical about the value of the arts and humanities in medicine than surgeons. Yet surgeons readily engage with music. Playing music in operating theatres is common practice, where many surgeons claim that music helps them to concentrate. Elmere Vize (2010), blogging about the beneficial use of music in operating theatres, says: "Music reduces stress. It lifts moods, making the operating room a more pleasant work environment". Such positive use of music is noted in a 1924 edition of the magazine *Popular Mechanics*:

> music has been found of value in surgical operations to ease patients during and after the administration of ether. Melodies are supplied by a phonograph or instrumental selections are rendered by an artist. Several demonstrations have been made at a Brooklyn, New York, hospital.
>
> (Ibid)

Dr Jonathan Katz (in Stetka 2017), a clinical professor of anesthesiology at Yale University School of Medicine, says: "The evidence suggests that carefully self-selected music can have a beneficial effect on some surgeons during specific stages of the surgery". However, a systematic review of 17 studies of the effect of music in the operating theatre (Vahed et al. 2016) showed that while surgeons said that they benefitted through focus of attention, communication between nurses and surgeons was sometimes hindered by music. Anaesthetists may resent intrusion on their technical auditory space, where they monitor sound signals. Music can provide an unwanted distraction. A 1997 study of 200 anaesthetists' views on music in the operating theatre showed that over a quarter felt that music was intrusive, reducing their vigilance and frustrating wider communication across the surgical team, and over a half found music distracting if they were trying to attend to an anaesthetic problem (Vize 2010). Writing anonymously in an online forum (Medscape), a surgeon commented: "I used to do music in the OR, but I began to find it distracting. I think it's become a badge of cool, and I am in favour of treating surgery seriously" (Stetka 2017). Again, here are the contested medical humanities in the wild – ambient arts in health care.

Noise is everywhere in hospitals, often irritating and unhelpful to sick or recovering patients and their anxious relatives and friends, as Tom Rice's (2013) formative book on medicine, sound and sonic alignment details. Stetka (2017) notes: "noise levels in operating rooms can exceed 120 decibels, louder than a busy highway". In orthopaedic theatres, where drilling is common, noise levels can be higher. One would think that playing music would only add to the cacophany. I have already noted how high levels of ambient noise – such as traffic and machinery – in general constitute a major public health hazard.

A Pennsylvania surgeon Dr Evan O'Neil Kane first took a gramophone into the operating room in 1914 on the basis that playing soothing music would help patients relax prior to anaesthesia. An article in the *British Journal of Surgery* from 1995 – 'Music in the Operating Theatre' – suggested that levels of stress amongst staff and conscious patients (having surgery under a local anaesthetic) was reduced by music. But 'whose music?' is the key question. All the examples of 'relaxing' music in this 1995 article were classical, but surgeons now are more likely to play rock or pop music.

Research conducted at Imperial College London with the Institute of Education (Hofkins 2018) using videotape of 20 operations (14 of which had music playing) suggested that music in theatre does have its problems, especially if it is 'foreground' rather than 'background' where it can hinder attention of operating theatre nursing staff (scrub nurse, runner), and confound communication between surgeons and nurses, while it may help the concentration of surgeons. This research suggested that whether or not music should be played and choice of music genre should be ironed out in the compulsory briefing period before lists. The researchers found that around 70% of operations have music playing in theatres, ranging across all genres from classical to heavy metal.

Enriching practice through the arts

Let us return to value of the medical humanities in educating the sense of hearing to deepen it to a diagnostic 'listening'. There is a strong tradition of music *as* medicine, as an arts therapy, with a dedicated peer-reviewed journal *Music and Medicine*, and medical students could be made aware of this work, as it includes, for example, music in hospitals and research on how music affects the mind and body (see, e.g., McMaster Institute for Music and the Mind: https://mimm.mcmaster.ca).

But music *in* medicine is my concern here, or rather auditory culture meeting medical education – a world of practice that is described as 'sonic alignment' (Vannini et al. 2010; Rice 2013), where sounds are treated as activities that mix with other activities such as clinical practices and emotional responses. As sounds, practices and responses are brought together meaningfully, as in auscultation, for example, so 'sonic alignment' is achieved. This embodied approach to listening begins with treating the body as both instrument and soundscape affording diagnostic cues, and considers clinical environments as sonic spaces affording both healing and discomfort. Medical students who already play instruments will readily appreciate that the body can be 'played' as in percussion and auscultation, and that rhythm and improvisation are key elements in a doctor's repertoire.

Tm Dornan and Martina Kelly (2018: unpaginated), in championing links between music and medicine, refer to "a sensescape of healing" arising from a doctor's mindfulness linking what is nourishing about music and how patients can be nourished by the presence of a caring doctor. They stress how this shifts the basis of medicine from the functional to the existential. First, the musician and her audience can be compared to the doctor and her patient, invoking "bi-directional communication". Second, music, like medicine, obviously engages the senses, and can help medical students to develop auditory skills. Third and finally, music can help to encourage existential reflection – states of being and authenticity that may feed back into empathy with suffering persons. This focuses on 'being with' patients rather than doing things to them, where

> ... expert clinicians assimilate sight, sound, smell and touch into an integrated experience of patients' illnesses. This includes the patient's posture, facial expression, sound of breathing and pulse. Their proficient physical examinations are co-ordinated and smooth – their physical responses to their patients are orchestrated movements of body and mind as a form of bodily understanding.
>
> (Ibid)

Such clinical 'sonic alignment' deepens a series of events into an experience – in medicine, again to turn ordinary hearing into diagnostic listening and to reject objectification of patients for dialogical care. A typical case of alignment, say in auscultation, occurs between (i) what is heard via the stethoscope as the sonics of the patient's body (score); (ii) what goes on in the head of the medical student or doctor in terms of recognition of this sound in relation to a register (an imagination of symptoms such as use of metaphors as similes – 'sounds like Velcro being pulled open') (sight reading of the score); (iii) what goes on in the way of touch and conversation between medical student or doctor and patient, in building a therapeutic alliance during the consultation (orchestrated movements); and (iv) what emotional responses are called forth in both doctor and patient (improvised passages).

A fifth element can be added – that of processional practice. Here, medical students call on knowledge of the history of, for example, mediate auscultation in placing themselves in this historical stream – from which an identity emerges (as identification with a community of practice). As agents in an expanding activity system or community of practice (medicine), generations of doctors do not just reproduce what went before but creatively re-imagine and invent, opening up new objects of inquiry and new horizons of research.

Percussion and auscultation both combine an imaginative art and humanity of close noticing with the sciences of anatomy and physiology. Such humanity has been stressed in the previous chapter. Listening to the patient through percussion and auscultation – treating the body imaginatively as a sonic instrument and its interior as a soundscape – demands being close to patients. The therapeutic relationship is again key. Some architectural imagination is necessary as the body's interior architecture is sensed within clinical spaces where sound can often act as distraction and irritant, even pollution, such as the ambient sound of busy hospital wards – although experienced doctors claim that such sounds merely become wallpaper and do not create a distraction. Again, one wonders what happens to the repression of feelings associated with irritant ambient sound? Does such repressed affect return in a distorted form? Such an admittance that background noise becomes like 'wallpaper' suggests not just innocuous habit and saturation through exposure, but rather production of insensibility, an an-aesthetising – a little like forgetting to water the plant in your office or on your desk, only to notice one day that it has withered and died. The dying, pot-bound, un-watered and un-nourished plant can become a symbol for the growing cynicism of the doctor and that doctor's psychological and physical state on the burnout curve. Let's nourish the doctor as we would want to save the plant.

Against this background of factors, the art of listening can be deepened in many ways while enhancing, rather than detracting from, the medicine and surgery curriculum. This might be summarised as an education for 'music related sensibility'.

Ten examples of 'sonic alignment' embodied learning or body pedagogics

Clinical connections

Every hospital will have an audiology department and students can ask for placements here to see the creative ways in which sound is used. The hospital in which my own medical school is situated has a very creative paediatric audiology department. This has been purpose-designed with equipment such as videotape facilities to allow audiologists, child psychologists, sensory support teams and parents to watch replays of how they interact with their children with hearing difficulties, and, importantly, to watch how parents interact with each other in communicating with, say, their profoundly deaf child. Eye, Nose and Throat (ENT) surgeons may also be involved in these activities where a child is scheduled for surgery. The department also draws on use of drama experts to help parents to improve communication with deaf children.

A key related issue is that of the medicalisation of deafness. A more radical, politicised deaf community resists framing deafness as a disability that must be attended to medically. The sharp end of this is the debate about the value of cochlear implant technologies (Moir and Overy 2014). The majority of people who have had cochlear implants complain that their hearing of music is greatly compromised. Topics such as these invite study through the lenses of the medical humanities.

'Available' music environments in medical schools

Sometimes, debates about introducing medical humanities into undergraduate medicine and surgery curricula miss what is right under our noses. Many doctors play instruments, many medical schools have bands, orchestras and choirs, and many have music-based arts projects for patients on the wards, or at a minimum a hospital radio service. Students will then have ready-made contexts to keep up their interests in music. For example, Dalhousie University Medical School in Halifax, Nova Scotia, has a world-renowned 'music in medicine' programme with an in-house ('Tupper') band established for 40 years (www.dal.ca/news/today/2016/08/08/medical_humanities_music_in_medicine_program.html).

Creating an academic culture through high profile appointments and building on existing faculty interests

Setting up a dedicated community of practice based around educating hearing to develop diagnostic listening may require the injection of high-profile faculty. At Peninsula Medical School, we realised that developing a core, integrated and assessed medical humanities programme starts with faculty development. We sought judicious use of ambient talent, so that, for example, physicians with musical interest and expertise were eager to teach students clinical listening skills. A community of practice can be seeded where music is common talk and this spills over into clinical learning. This facilitates intersubjective learning and creates an atmosphere and ecology that affords learning, where students are infected with a passion for pedagogy. The current Vice-Dean for Education at my medical school is an experienced general practitioner and medical educator, but is also a bass player in a punk rock band (his son plays drums in the same band). It is easy for him to offer analogies for medical students between medicine and music. He runs a medical humanities Special Studies Unit called 'School of Rock', where a small group of students form a band and have an opportunity to write music, and rehearse and play in a professional studio setting, producing a CD that is sold for charity. They then perform at a student-led conference. But the students in the band do not just play music – they also debate and reflect upon issues raised in this chapter about connections between music and medicine, especially teamwork, 'hitting the right note', and establishing rhythms at work.

A doctor and medical educator, Paul Haidet, has for over a decade used jazz to show his students how to improvise in the medical encounter, both literally (Haidet 2007) and as a metaphor (Haidet et al. 2017), developing a course for medical students (Sayani 2010). Typically, students would work on similarities between communication with patients and playing jazz, including quality of talk such as 'phrasing', improvising, leaving space and call-and-response.

At Peninsula Medical School, we were lucky enough to appoint the late Paul Robertson (a virtuoso violinist and educationalist and leader of the famed string quartet the Medici Quartet) as Visiting Professor of Music and Medicine, while one of our Vice-Deans (now retired), Professor Tony Pinching, also a consultant physician, is a passionate musician and composer. Both provided talks and a collaborative longitudinal Special Study Unit on music and medicine. Following on from a long-established 'peripatetic ethics' expert (he called himself the 'roaming ethicist') – an anaesthetist who provided input on ethical issues on ward rounds and in surgery with groups of students – we wanted to provide a peripatetic musician who could join ward rounds, talking to the students about the influence of sound in the hospital. But this never materialised, as Paul Robertson tragically died in the wake of an aortic rupture from which he at first recovered and then relapsed. He told his story of 'death in life' while in a state of suspension in critical care in a poignant memoir (Robertson 2016).

Paul Robertson worked closely with students on the value of studying how music is played with others (e.g., in his world class string quartet) as a model for clinical teamwork. Fruitful comparisons can be made between the way that a string quartet or a jazz quartet move between written music and improvisation, and a clinical team, such as a surgical team, work in real time (partly scripted, partly improvised). In my own work researching surgical teamwork and developing surgical education, teams watched videos of jazz groups performing and tracked how close listening allowed for switches between players as they played common themes and bridges, and then improvised solos. These advertise issues such as 'timing', 'handovers' and how 'leadership' and 'followership' can emerge in fluid team dynamics.

Resulting from running the Special Study Unit in Music and Medicine for fourth year medical students, Robertson (2014) offers a rationale not, as might be expected, for the integration of music into undergraduate medical education, but rather for the recognition of 'thinking with music' and 'appreciating through music' as implicit resources. Students would repeatedly find that music had woven its way into their ways of thinking and imagining. It was not difficult to get them to think creatively about clinical work in terms of, say, rhythm and melody, composition and performance, timbre, resonance and dissonance and so forth. At a minimum, students would take away the notion that their embodied practices exhibited both volume and tone controls. How would they use these in encounters with both patients and colleagues?

Interdisciplinary activities within institutions should be encouraged – medical schools can collaborate with music departments. A good example of this in the UK is the collaboration between Professors Roger Kneebone and Aaron Williamon. Kneebone, introduced in earlier chapters, is a Professor of surgical education, and a surgeon who has also worked as a General Practitioner. He and Williamon co-direct the Royal College of Music (RCM) – Imperial College (University of London) Centre for Performance Science (http://performancescience.ac.uk), launched in 2016. Williamon is Professor at the Royal College of Music, London and has a dual background in music and psychology. The Centre's interest is Performance Studies. Kneebone is the UK's leading expert in interdisciplinary work across arts, crafts, performance and surgery (that feeds in to a Masters course in surgical education). Typically, a study area might be 'manual dexterity', where a range of high performance skills such as tailoring, music and stitching wounds in medicine and surgery are considered for mutual learning and emergent pedagogies. Opportunities will probably abound for such collaborations but may not yet have been investigated.

Also, Maastrict University has a renowned 'Sonic Skills' interdisciplinary research project that focuses on 'listening for knowledge in science, medicine and engineering' (https://cris.maastrichtuniversity.nl/portal/en/publications/sonic-skills(da32067c-9898-461a-87ab-e5a81b5ce56d).html).

Specific skills: (i) 'ear cleaning'

During the 1960s, the famous American cardiologist W Proctor Harvey introduced 'ear cleaning' into teaching auscultation to both medical students and postgraduates (March 2002). Harvey would play a recording of Beethoven's Symphony No. 9 as the audience came into the room and would then question them about hearing specific instruments such as the French horn, piano, violin and kettle drum. Students invariably say that they did not, on 'casual' listening, pick out a particular instrument. Harvey would then deepen 'casual' listening to focused hearing, educating the ear by listening specifically for named instruments, discriminating between tones. Of course, the audience finds this relatively easy. Harvey then transfers this across to auscultation, using the same principle, the gestalt of figure and ground, claiming transfer of organising principles.

At first, all is ground to students, but, as they identify particular instruments and bring them forward as figures, so a vigilant attention kicks in as the paradoxical attention of constant sound scanning continues. Acute (vigilant) attentive hearing plays against chronic (paradoxical) attentive hearing. The students learn both deep listening and agile listening as similes (such as a polyphonic orchestration of heart sounds, where the skill is to foreground specific diagnostic sounds). Just as the sound source is collective (although within one body), so the listening can be collective and collaborative, amongst a body of students working as a co-educating audience, creating connoisseurship.

Contemporary students may or may not balk at Beethoven. Certainly there are imaginative options such as the San Franciscan duo Matmos, who incorporate everyday sounds into electronic music such as unwrapping food items, to sounds garnered from liposuction (https://vimeo.com/300506148) and human blood flow (www.soundonsound.com/people/matmos). Matthew Herbert also uses everyday sounds. His album 'A Nude (The Perfect Body)' (https://soundcloud.com/accidentalrecords-1/sets/a-nude-the-perfect-body-by) could offer an intriguing supplement for anatomy learning. Herbert's electronic sound piece is conceived as a sonic nude, rather than an illustrated or painted nude. Body sounds create imaginative connections that clearly illustrate the complexities of an embodied and phenomenological approach to experience. Tracks include improvisations on sound connected with the body: grooming, sleeping, waking, shitting, hurting, eating, moving and 'coming'.

Medical students could be set a task of working with an electronic musician to produce a Matmos or Matthew Herbert type of music based on a 'starter vocabulary', such as the contrast between normal resonant sounds over the lungs and hyperresonance over hollows such as the bowel and pneumothorax, with dull normal and abnormal sounds over the liver or consolidated area of lung, and stony dull sounds over fluid filled areas such as in a pleural effusion. This could also be disseminated as an educational resource and used for public engagement.

One of our fourth year medical students produced a sound piece with a written critical commentary for a Special Study Unit based on the junior doctors' strikes in the UK of 2017–18. The piece mixed electronics with sound clips taken from live recordings of marches and demonstrations during the strike. It offers a powerful memento of a key era in the politicising of doctors in the UK as they fought primarily to protect the National Health Service (NHS) from creeping privatisation promoted by a Tory government, as well as protesting their own work and pay conditions.

Specific skills: (ii) phenomenology of 'in head' listening

Medical students are used to 'in head' listening, having grown up with mobile phones with music capabilities. Stethoscopes feel different to ear-bud headphones and require a new 'in head' normalisation. 'In head' listening, rather than naturalistic or 'open space' listening, affords a site for "cultural techniques of listening" (Stankievech 2007: 56). Charles Stankievech (2007) opens our imagination to listening with the stethoscope not as a purely instrumental activity but as an aesthetic event, a performance and an art. We must read medical listening as a cultural event beyond the literal and instrumental. This is reinforced by the fact that listening to signs and symptoms is mediated linguistically (particularly through similes or resemblances), and that the mapping of signs is not an objective process.

There is significant variation amongst a group of experienced clinicians in how a common heart, lung or digestive sound is heard. Stankievech describes stethoscopic listening phenomenologically – how an individual experiences 'in head' listening and how discrimination is formed. This involves both what is listened to and how this listening is simultaneously explored and given meaning; or appears meaningless, confusing or irritating. Pure sound is mixed with cognitive and emotional responses within the same spatial arrangement. In short, without tuition, 'in head' listening can remain at the level of 'event' prior to becoming an experience.

Despite the yearning for standardised assessments across clinical skills examinations, when it comes to experienced practice, doctors hear the same lung and heart sounds differently, according to personal style. Yet they can readily correspond in diagnoses. Musicians similarly play a common written score with differing outcomes partly because of their idiosyncracies across 'in head' listening. Performing sound in medicine invites individual style rather than conformity and standardisation.

Practice, practice, practice

The well-known joke told earlier refers to a musician carrying a violin case who asks a passerby 'how do I get to Carnegie Hall?' The passerby says: 'Practice, practice, practice!' Medical students learning percussion and auscultation must practice, practice, practice! But this can be enhanced. First, collaborative practice is essential. Like playing in a small group or in a larger group and then an orchestra, your own musical sensibility or perception is afforded by the quality of the music environment around you. It is enhanced through collaboration, feedback and mutual learning.

While students practice, again why not bring in a tabla player (a fingertip and percussion expert) to work with the group to educate the fingertips and wrist action for percussive techniques (and, as a sideline, learning how the heartbeat may be translated from lub-dup into tak-dina-din)?

Learning from anthropology

An anthropological sensibility helps us to revision our native environments. While Western culture is oriented to the visual, there are cultures, for example, living in dense jungle, that are primarily oriented to the acoustic. Medical students might study some anthropological examples of such cultures not for their local medical lore but for their sonic worldview. The term 'sonic alignment' was coined by anthropologists (Vannini et al. 2010) and refers to a performative process of ordering meanings in sound. For example, surgeons do not just blithely choose music to play in the operating theatre – it is a statement of power and identity. They might even 'conduct' a particularly difficult operation through gestural breathing – as with an orchestra's conductor, upward motions for inspiration and downward diminuendo for expiration and concentration.

Working solely with a compendium of analogies

There is so much mileage in exploring metaphors ('a rasping cough') and analogies ('a crackling like the sound of cellophane being scrunched'). The medical imagination is part sensory, part semantic (linguistic-literary) and part scientific (anatomy, physiology and biochemistry knowledge). A sense impression is shaped diagnostically by a known metaphor and an underpinning scientific explanation. For example, where a normal heart sound can be likened to a flowing river, a heart murmur sounds like a rocky river (Pick 2013). As Roger Kneebone's (www.imperial.ac.uk/people/r.kneebone) body of work shows, referred to throughout this book, the benefits from interdisciplinary comparisons and collaborations are not additive but multiplicative.

Some of the fruitful comparisons across medicine and traditional skill/ craft/apprenticeship trades are surprising. For example, Stefan Krebs and Melissa Van Drie (2014) compare listening practices of doctors and car mechanics (often called 'auto doctors'). Expert car mechanics can hear minor changes in pitch in engine sounds – indicating the need for 'tuning' – that are inaudible to novices. The engine is treated as musical instrument. Just as medical imaging has displaced auscultation, so oscilloscopes have replaced the educated ear of the car mechanic. In both cases, the culturally dominant ocular has prevailed. Just as deep knowledge of auscultation's litany of metaphors (analogies and resemblances) formed a basis for the identity construction of the doctor, so the 'auto doctor' will be defined in the future in the absence of direct listening.

Cross-discipline: drawings

That the arts are integral to learning clinical medicine is readily advertised by teaching students sense-based techniques, such as percussion and auscultation, through linking listening and touch with drawing. Physical examination textbooks characteristically ask students to sketch a chest surface anatomy and label with points where they would listen, for example, for each valve (tricuspid, pulmonic, mitral, aortic) and for murmurs (aortic stenosis, pulmonic stenosis, mitral regurgitation, tricuspid regurgitation, aortic regurgitation, mitral stenosis). Use of colours can group murmurs (systolic and diastolic); shade of colour could indicate when in the cycle (e.g., mid-systolic vs pansystolic); depth of colour could indicate pitch, intensity and quality. A 'B' or 'D' could indicate whether the sound is best heard with the bell or diaphragm of the stethoscope. Arrows could indicate possible radiations. Better, students can work on each other or on standardised patients, sketching directly on to the chest where appropriate. A visual vocabulary is then built up to augment and act as mnemonic for the auditory.

Studying sound artists

An example of how a compulsory mis-education can produce insensibility in medical students happened in my own medical school in clinical skills training for communication. The good news was that nurses ran the clinical skills centres across three locations, and nurses are usually good at listening and teaching others how to listen. The deep listening skills of psychotherapists and counsellors were unfortunately not drawn on to teach communication – a mistake in curriculum planning. The nurses, however, had to work with a standardised, pragmatic and formulaic 'professional' communication package, where students practiced with actor patients. This stultified and distorted learning communication for many students, both stifling their 'natural' abilities and displaying problems of transfer to authentic clinical contexts – although some students liked the structure and the opportunity to 'fail safely'. While simulation learning for interventionist clinical skills makes sense for patient safety reasons, learning clinical communication in simulated settings has its problems (Bleakley et al. 2011).

We appointed a Visiting Professor of Visual Art, Christine Borland (2006), an established artist who was a Turner Prize finalist and one of the original Young British Artists (YBA) group. Christine focused on simulation training in clinical skills to produce a series of works that were formally curated as a public engagement show at the Newlyn Art Gallery in Penzance, UK. In one of the works, Christine Borland interviewed several Years 3 and 4 medical students about the value of communication skills training, and recorded the interviews. Many, again, felt that the clinical skills 'professional' communication courses were forced, stifling natural ability and often ineffective and counterproductive, as when they met real patients they had to improvise in sometimes challenging and often unpredictable contexts.

The recorded interviews – often critical then of the teaching methods – were played back through a number of small speakers attached to the back of a large white screen. At the front of the screen, several stethoscopes were hung for the public to use. Somebody was at hand to help them to use the stethoscope properly (bell or diaphragm) if they wished, but they were encouraged to experiment. Also, student helpers could show the public how to percuss the board to discover the duller sounds where the speakers were attached. Members of the public would then search across the front of the board as if carrying out a physical examination, and would eventually pass over one of the speakers, where a student would be talking about the issues of translating a taught, standardised method as opposed to relying on their natural listening capabilities.

In defence of teaching clinical skills this way, medical educators will tell you that some students are very poor communicators and do need a structured method and practice (where they can get feedback). Also, sensitive issues such as breaking bad news do need practice with feedback. However, one should ask why students are admitted to a medical course in the first place if they are poor communicators. The point of the example is that an artist can bring a new angle on a medical education issue, to encourage us to 'think otherwise' about that issue. Working with an artist such as Christine Borland also inspired students to study other artists working with medical themes. In the area of listening, this includes Linda Montano's 'Heart Murmur' from 1975, where she taped a stethoscope to her body for a week, living in a gallery, to exorcise what she described as a 'broken heart' that only art could save (Stankievech 2007).

There are many body-related sound pieces by performance artists that medical students may benefit from studying, such as *Crackers* by Christof Migone. Migone advertised for volunteers who could 'crack' joints (knuckles are the most common). The cracking was then sound recorded and disseminated as a MP3 file, or videotaped with sound and presented as a film projection. Migone (2002: unpaginated) extends the individual cracking sounds to a multiple 'crackerscape'. This extends the metaphor of 'cracking' twinned with the real sounds of joints cracking, as

> ... a portrait of a city through the cracking bones of its citizens. This is a specific form of soundscape, it is a crackerscape. The portraits feature forms of behavior that navigate nervously between the controllable and the uncontrollable. A city's identity contains an inherent tension between order and chaos. ... The individual contains similar internal struggles. ... a joint is the locale where bones articulate a tension. Crackers are compulsive about the release of that tension. As the sound of the cracks echo, some wince, others feel relief. In all instances, a crack is when and where something breaks.

Such art-based approaches can make us 'think otherwise' about anatomy, orthopaedic surgery and rheumatology, offering rich, complex and interesting resources for getting at the human face of, say, rheumatoid arthritis – its existential as well as medical nature.

Hearing and listening as communication expertise

I have purposely kept the most obvious area of 'listening' in medicine – the doctor listening to the patient in a consultation – to the end of this chapter, and I will keep this brief. This is because there is a very large literature in this area – I have written extensively on this myself (for example, Bleakley 2014). William Osler, the father of modern medicine, advised his students: "Just listen to your patient; he is telling you the diagnosis". But a consistent body of evidence shows that doctors hear, but are not great listeners. On average, doctors interrupt their patients 11 seconds into the consultation (Ospina et al. 2019). Further, as the consultation continues, doctors talk more than their patients (Ofri 2017). There may be an adequate functional explanation for this – doctors are pressed for time, and so may hurry the patient on to get as much information as they can in the time allotted. But also, doctors may not have learned impulse control and the tendency to interrupt; and further, might tune out the patient's voice as they turn instead to care protocols and electronic health records.

All of this is worrying as another body of evidence indicates the health benefits of good communication between doctors and patients (Ha and Longnecker 2010). Paradoxically, as psychotherapists and psychoanalysts will tell you, intensive listening actually tends to lead to more information as well as emotional or cathartic release from the client or patient, than interruption. So interrupting, even for purposes of clarification, may be a clumsy intervention in what is the demanding and defined professional social context of the consultation.

Further, doctors overestimate their abilities to listen well (ibid), while communication skills can deteriorate over time in a doctor's career, as cynicism may grow: "The emotional and physical brutality of medical training ... suppresses empathy, substitutes techniques and procedures for talk, and may even result in derision for patients". Doctors are simply not taught to listen well. Indeed, paradoxically, recent research data (Moral et al. 2019: 55) "suggest that students' attitudes toward CS (communication skills) could decline as a result of CS training".

Moral et al. suggest that "Learning CS with experiential methods seems to be challenging for students at a personal level" (ibid). Communication 'training' (of 'skills' and not capabilities) suffers from reduction to instrumental protocols and, unless a medical student goes into psychiatry or general practice as a specialty, there is little opportunity to develop expertise as listeners. In contrast, an education as a psychotherapist requires the gaining of expertise as a multi-layered capability involving (i) the exercise of vigilant and paradoxical attention, (ii) close listening as a 'listening through' to what is just below the surface of what the client (patient) says and (iii) checking the congruence between what is said (the verbal) and what is 'given off' (the non-verbal), where what is said often mis-directs or occludes. This suggests that medical students could benefit from learning professional communication from psychotherapists, and certainly should be offered therapeutic supervision during their education. They would further benefit from learning a collaborative self-help listening technique such as co-counselling (Heron 1974).

As noted earlier, Paul Haidet developed a way of teaching listening to medical students based on listening to jazz and jazz performance (see in particular Sayani 2010). For example, students are introduced to "Mastering Space": "For the next two weeks, pick one time when the patient is finishing a sentence. Wait for at least 10 seconds before saying anything. If the patient talks before 10 seconds, follow up on what they say". A second exercise is "Cultivating Ensemble": "For the next two weeks, say a sentence that begins with: 'So what I'm hearing you say is ...'. Do this with every patient". In working with communication between nurses and surgeons in operating theatre teams, I have successfully translated both these exercises as ways of getting surgeons to dialogue with team members rather than fall into habitual monologue. For context, we watched a film of contemporary jazz musicians playing in small group (quartet and quintet) and analysed the way that "cultivating ensemble" interlaced with improvised solos.

In summary, here are what I see as medical education's self-inflicted issues with educating for listening:

1   Medical schools continue to recruit students who show lack of agreeable sociability. In fact, too many students turn out to be chronically poor at communicating with others in a democratic manner: skilled at listening, turn taking, empathic response and emotional sensitivity – or, again, "cultivating ensemble".

2   Senior doctors tend to role model telling, informing and confronting (monological communication) rather than showing capability for supporting, engaging positively with another's emotional responses and feeling comfortable with discussion and question and answer rather than compulsively resorting to telling (dialogical communication). Inflexible hierarchical rather than democratic institutional structures reinforce such patterns of communication.

3   Related to point 2 is the socialisation of medical students into a culture of inflation (Bleakley 2020a), especially with male students. Here, medical students and doctors may overestimate their abilities including the ability to listen well, as noted above.

4   Communication is too heavily 'professionalised', or framed as idiosyncratic, where it could be re-aligned with more 'natural' and habitual ways in which medical students communicate in their everyday lives. For example, 'breaking bad news' and communicating during intimate examinations have been medicalised – treated as if they were 'hospital acquired specialties', where they are facts of everyday life and could be educated as such on the basis of shared social experiences.

5   Communication is turned into a package of 'skills' and often taught in a formulaic and structured, linear manner. In fact, communication 'in the wild' is sometimes chaotic and unstructured, and certainly partial and full of 'noise' as well as 'information'. Teaching and learning such structured communication is usually formally offered in the clinical skills curriculum and setting, where it is confounded by simulation, especially the use of standardised (actor) 'patients' working from standardised scripts and scenarios (for purposes of fairness in assessment). Simulation learning does not transfer well to real life contexts where there are no 'standard' patients or colleagues.

6   In the ideal setting of clinical work-based learning, communication (such as working in team settings as well as, say, bedside encounters with patients), learning communication is often ad hoc and unstructured. Ideally, there should be briefing, structured learning with feedback and then debriefing where 'communication' and 'clinical knowledge' including acquiring capability in diagnostic reasoning, are not separated out.

Medical education may then, certainly in part, be providing another unintended consequence – a compulsory mis-education in listening and hearing. Again, if such an education were successful, we would not have such a high incidence of two forms of error down the line. First, the ongoing 'crooked timber' in the institutional structure of medicine and surgery that is the early interruption of patients and the dominance of talk by doctors in the consultation, linked with the lack of insight, particularly with male doctors, into how well they do communicate (overestimation of capability being the norm). Second – especially in surgical settings – the (heavily documented) relatively high incidence of medical error arising from poor communication within and between clinical teams.

Jerome Groopman (2007), amongst others, notes how poor communication, especially listening, can lead to misdiagnoses, 'tuning out' the patient's voice. We can add to this the consistent finding that medical students and junior doctors are relatively poor at mediate auscultation, especially in differentiating heart sounds, even after reasonable exposure (Bernstein 2016). This is partly explicable by the inherent difficulty in skill and the lack of dedicated practice, but may also be explained by lack of attention to innovative teaching informed by theories of 'sonic alignment' for example, as detailed earlier.

Finally, but importantly, how much care do doctors take in cultivating speech? This is particularly important in the growing field of telephone consultations, where voice is the only input with patients. Choice of words, rhythm, diction and so forth are very important factors in communicating with patients. Medicine can be lyrical where mere information giving is not enough. Voice is core to care. Voice matters, so let us take more care over how we educate both voice and listening.

6 "How do I look?"

From 'looking' to 'seeing'

Thirty shades of white

After earlier Ancient Egyptian medical texts (2000–1500 BCE), the first recorded guides to clinical judgement in the visual realm can be found in Leviticus 13 in the Old Testament, written around 1440–1400 BC. It is a section entitled 'How leprosy is to be recognised':

> If the priest, looking at the place on his skin, finds that the hairs have turned white and the skin of the part affected seems shrunken compared with the rest of the skin around it, this is the scourge of leprosy .... If the skin is marked by a shiny white patch, but is not shrunken, and the hairs have kept their colour, the priest will shut him away for a week, and on the seventh day examine him .... If the priest finds a white swelling that has turned the hair white, and shows the raw, live flesh, then it must be pronounced leprosy inveterate, deeply rooted in the skin ...

Exegesis of this section by both medics and biblical scholars since the 19th century has noted that 'leprosy' (Hebrew *tsaraath*) probably refers to either vitiligo or the different disease of psoriasis. (Although vitiligo may be in the differential diagnosis for hypopigmented patches of leprosy.) Darla Schumm and Mchael Stoltzfus (2011) argue that *Leviticus* does differentiate between leprosy and vitiligo.

Rabbis identified over 30 shades of white in diagnosing this 'leprosy', drawing on a 'colour chart' of natural referents such as wool, snow, lime and "the membrane of an egg". The clinical judgement is grounded in the realm of the senses in the absence of any knowledge of the actual pathophysiological cause of the skin disorder(s). Of course, we have no record of how accurate this form of visual recognition of symptom proved to be, for example, of misdiagnoses (false positives and false negatives). But here we have the Rabbi's visual sense filtered through a preparatory cognitive map as probably the earliest recorded example of what we now call Type 1 reasoning, or 'intuitive' pattern recognition (as opposed to Type 2 reasoning or slower, deliberate cognitive reasoning based on logical decisions).

Such pattern recognition based on resemblance is not trivial – think again of the complexity and sophistication of the sense-based process of discriminating over 30 shades of white from natural referents from nearly 3,500 years ago (modern Pantone colour charts are only 50 years old). This is a colour palette discrimination you would expect from an experienced painter.

Here is a contemporary example of use of a tacit 'colour chart' in clinical reasoning, in this case by a nurse. Jane Cioffi (2000a: 266, 2000b, 2002), in a study of nurses' experiences in deciding to call for emergency assistance for patients, shows the importance of close sensory noticing of signs and symptoms: "You can tell by looking at someone … you pick up on the little things". One nurse says in the study of a patient: "The colour is not right … could be grayish not quite greyish as that is too far … more sallow, pallid" – taking us back to '30 shades of white'.

The renowned cultural commentator Walter Benjamin (2008/1936) noted: "the manner in which human sense perception is organised … is determined not only by nature but by historical circumstances as well". To 'historical' we must add 'cultural', for example, shifting attitudes towards body odours. In the subculture of medicine, as noted in previous chapters, the normal cultural education of disgust and revulsion must be suspended, for the sensory abject is everyday.

A dis-embodied road map for clinical reasoning – illness scripts learned *in vitro*

Abraham Verghese (1999: 299) warns against leading students too quickly into pattern recognition: "a blink-of-an-eye diagnosis" and trusting "the animal snout", for fear of misdiagnosing based on lack of experience and necessary connoisseurship. Medical students, early in their careers, must learn – from texts, lectures, small group work and limited clinical exposure (mostly ad hoc rather than providing scaffolded learning including briefing and debriefing) – to build 'illness scripts' (Custers 2015). These are road maps or blueprints for making a differential diagnosis on the basis of gathering evidence about presenting symptoms. They have been developed and refined over the past 30 years in medical education.

In utilising illness scripts, a set of presenting symptoms, contextualised in a broader clinical scenario (gender, age, previous history, life circumstance, diet, exercise, habits such as smoking, alcohol consumption and exposure to environmental toxicity), is distilled into oppositional pairs that form skeleton 'semantic qualifiers' such as acute/chronic, mild/severe and diffuse/localised. This points to predisposing conditions, disease manifestation and possible course of illness. Within these broad categories, elements such as epidemiology, time course, pathophysiology, salient symptoms and signs, diagnostics and possible treatments are identified. These broad areas are gradually laid down as 'cognitive illness scripts' in the doctor's memory, eventually providing a basis for growing confidence in pattern recognition.

In a classroom context, medical students can formulate a differential diagnosis through a worksheet, moving from gathering diagnostic evidence to problem representation to generating an illness script (Levin et al. 2016) – medicine under a bell jar.

An illness script for pneumonia acquired outside of a clinical setting such as a hospital (community acquired) looks like this:

Pathophysiology: infection of lower respiratory tract most commonly caused by *Streptococcus pneumoniae* (although fungal and viral infections cannot be ruled out).

Epidemiology: increased risk with age, structural lung disease, immunodeficiency and post-upper respiratory tract viral infection.

Time course: acute = days; progressively worsens if untreated.

Salient symptoms and signs: fever, shortness of breath, cough, tachycardia, hypoxemia, tachypnoea.

Diagnostics: labs and imaging: leucocytosis, bacteria in sputum or blood cultures, lobar infiltrate on chest X-ray.

Treatment: antibiotics.

There are riders to this formulaic approach. For example, both congestive heart failure and chronic obstructive pulmonary disease exacerbation resemble community-acquired pneumonia, but a lobar infiltrate on a chest X-ray without cardiomegaly (abnormal enlargement of the heart) or cephalization (dilation due to increased pressure) of vessels is highly suggestive of pneumonia and then makes congestive heart failure less likely. Also, in an elderly patient, there may be absence of fever while pneumonia remains the correct diagnosis.

Medical students learning this script *in vitro* are practising a disembodied medicine. *In vivo* the patient's symptoms impact on the senses; diagnostic work is embodied, vital and authentic. Illness scripts learned *in vitro* are abstract and purely linguistic, where an illness script is better performed *in vivo*, as sensate and where language becomes activity – a meaningful gesture at the bedside more vital than mental gymnastics in a simulation setting. 'Hothousing' or accelerating diagnostic acumen in medical students invites embodiment – engaging at the bedside in hospital for acute conditions and in the General Practice surgery for chronic conditions, where learning is purposefully scaffolded with briefing and de-briefing.

Illness scripts, useful – indeed indispensable – for physical illnesses, do not provide the same scaffolding possibilities when applied to psychological trauma. Indeed, in the face of violent embodiment of trauma, an illness script is merely a gesture, a ghost or an echo. To illustrate this, let us consider a highly embodied insult – aggressive or violent rape of a woman – that leaves a long-lasting psychological scar of post-traumatic stress, anxiety, distaste for the body, self-harming, generalised hatred for men and even suicidal thoughts or suicide attempts.

A woman is violently raped and is both too ashamed and sceptical that she will receive a hearing that she does not report this to the police (see Penner 2018 for 'the illness script of sexual assault'). For over a year, she re-lives the rape but does not seek help. Symptoms intensify – flashbacks, dreams, feelings of disgust, suicidal thoughts abound. Eventually, after admission to hospital for attempted suicide, she is offered psychiatric help. But her health insurers add insult to injury – this is a North American case – refusing to cover for fees, claiming that she has already coped for over a year, so why can this process of resilience not continue?

How will this be represented as an 'illness script' for the purposes of teaching? Each rape is uniquely insulting. Yes, there may be a symptom pattern for post-traumatic stress, but this too unfolds in unique ways. The raped woman is like a palimpsest – a manuscript page where the original text has been scraped off and a new one imposed from another document, a text that itself cannot be washed off. The point for this book's theme is that the insult of the rape is an assault on the senses that can lead to a radical de-sensualising, a numbing and a loss of quality of life. For the practitioner (a psychiatrist, clinical psychologist or psychotherapist) treating this woman, how will her tender psyche and now armoured body be approached without adding further insult? The conversations and interventions must be highly attuned sensually but without a hint of bodily insult that is now the woman's tangled and bruised emotional capital. The clinician's words must offer the lightest of touches for it is the heavy hand that delivered the abuse. And will the clinician be a woman, as reason suggests?

Will the clinician be able to translate the Levitican text that opens this chapter into the psychological realm? (A survey of 1,000 general practitioners in the UK shows that 40% of appointments are about mental health (Mind 2018).) Again, "If the priest finds a white swelling that has turned the hair white, and shows the raw, live flesh, then it must be pronounced leprosy inveterate, deeply rooted in the skin ...". The mental scar of rape is just as deeply embodied and rooted and when touched will be highly sensitive. Doctors forget that their words are like hands, sometimes inappropriately withdrawn or stilted in delivery, or over-abundant and suffocating the patient (a doctor who talks too much and fails to listen is promoting insensibility).

Embodied words

The anthropologist Franz Boas claimed that the 'Eskimos' have many words to describe different kinds of snow. Boas studied Inuit peoples on Baffin Island in Canada in the 1880s, where his 1911 *Handbook of American Indian Languages* suggested that the indigenous populations might have hundreds of words for 'snow', discriminating between types such as 'softly falling' and 'good for riding a sled'. This observation was later derided as an urban myth, but in fact Boas was correct. While Boas studied Inuit language, this is often conflated with Yupik, and when the two languages collide they produce a rich vocabulary to suggest that the sensory discrimination of types of snow does indeed describe 40–50 kinds, including snow that looks like salt, wet snow that ices quickly and so forth. Discrimination of differing types of sea ice embraces up to 70 types. This range is paltry compared with the Sami in modern Norway. An article (www.thelocal.no/20170421/reindeer-at-risk-from-arctic-hot-spell) describing *Norway's reindeer at risk from Arctic hot spell* claims:

> One of the Sami dialects counts no fewer than 318 words to describe different types of snow. "Seanas", for example, means a kind of grainy snow ideal for reindeer, making it easy for them to dig out the lichen and moss with their hooves.

While the Levitican example that opens this chapter is visual, here is an inter-sensory example engaging sight and touch, expanded by embodied metaphors or thinking-in-the-flesh (Lakoff and Johnson 1999).

These examples remind us of the link between what we sense and how we sense, and where discrimination operates. They also say much about achieving connoisseurship as a lived experience. The environment presents a multitude of sensory experiences, and we come to engage with these, and classify them, through language. The richer (more sensual) the language, informed by a poetic imagination, the closer we get to the environmental cues that afford an experience. This rule of thumb applies to medical diagnostics. While illness scripts collapse complex presentations into linear and simpler categories – for ease of memorisation – we see how this approach collapses in the psychological realm with the example of the woman who was raped, where an 'illness script' becomes an oxymoron. Here, we have a poetic, albeit highly disturbing, narrative reflecting the unique.

Over 1,500 years after Leviticus, the 'father' of medicine, Galen (AD 130–210) described how a doctor should watch how the patient moves, closely observe skin colour and take the pulse of the patient and touch him or her to determine body temperature; a rumbling stomach must be attended to closely to distinguish the type of rumbling as a diagnostic cue and clue; the patient's breath must be smelt; also the faeces, where the odours are again a diagnostic wellspring; while the patient's sweat or urine might also be tasted (Bynum and Porter 2004).

Islamic medicine too emphasised use of all the senses in diagnostic work. Over 1,500 years after the Levitican description of diagnosis of 'leprosy' was written, Ali Ibn Ridwan (c. 988–1061), an Egyptian scholar, suggests: "For your diagnosis ... you should always choose things that are extremely powerful and easy to recognise, and these are what can be perceived by sight, touch, hearing, smell, taste and by the intellect". A millennium later, contemporary medical students are in danger of losing these sense-based capacities for examination and diagnosis as direct sense-based diagnosis is being replaced by indirect or remote methods through technological extensions to the senses. Of course, such technologies enhance diagnostic acumen, but as repeated throughout this book, potentially at a cost. Will the future medical student know her vocabulary of 'shades of white' and 'types of snow' – a handbook of resemblances – as well as the Levitican priest or snow-dweller, or does this matter?

Educating the senses for diagnostic acumen: Type 1 reasoning

Medical students inevitably learn to diagnose from second-hand stories of their seniors, from textbooks and from simulated actor-patients in clinical skills 'laboratories'. Under these early learning circumstances, clinical reasoning follows a logical pattern where key presenting symptoms offer a differential diagnosis – a possibility of several underlying diseases that may only be narrowed down through further testing or imaging, or calling on an expert second opinion (for an overview, see Balogh et al. 2015). Students learn to work with 'decision trees' or an equivalent – formulaic ways of rationally narrowing down diagnostic options. This kind of rational, linear reasoning is called 'Type 2'. We met this earlier in the form of 'illness scripts' with associated 'semantic qualifiers' such as acute/chronic. I described this as a kind of necessary educational sterility, but one that must be given flavour – or rather fleshed out – by early and repeated exposure to live clinical work, with appropriate educational support (scaffolding, briefing and debriefing – the holy trinity of good work-based pedagogy).

As students become trainee doctors, full working professionals and specialists in a medical or surgical field, so their expertise naturally develops and becomes focused. In this process, 'Type 1' clinical reasoning gradually replaces 'Type 2' as the default mode. Here, the evidence of the senses is primary, as rapid, 'intuitive' decisions based on familiar presenting patterns of symptom are brought into play and can be trusted ("the animal snout"). The exception to this is a rare disease or a previously unseen configuration. This has been likened to an expert detective's use of cues and clues that would not be observed by the layperson or the novice, but present to the expert as a recognisable pattern (Hunter 1991). This is not just occult medical knowledge: the public too know about 'sleuthing' in medicine from the television medical soap opera 'House MD', where Gregory House, played by Hugh Laurie, is scripted as obnoxious, prickly, opioid-addicted and mildly autistic, but is a brilliant diagnostician. His relationship with patients is summed up as follows: "if you can fake sincerity, you can fake pretty much anything" and "it's a basic truth of the human condition that everybody lies". House MD was the most watched television programme worldwide in

2008 and consistently in the top 10 in America 2004–12. Precisely what does the public imagination make of this?

The anatomy of Type 1 clinical reasoning, or pattern recognition, still remains somewhat a mystery to experts, and it is unclear how much Type 1 reasoning can be 'hothoused' or accelerated through medical education of novices or early career doctors with growing expertise. Certainly, we can be sure that there is a link between education of the senses and development of clinical judgement acumen, but medical education leaves much of this to chance in the context of a traditional apprenticeship of learning on the job. Much more can be done in the way of structuring medical education to promote 'hothousing' of clinical reasoning. This depends first on anatomising the links between sense and judgement, and second on developing an informed medical pedagogy – optimising conditions under which learning to use the senses can be accelerated. Here, the medical humanities can play a central role.

For example, a professional visual artist is an expert in visual acumen and may have undergone up to a decade of formal education and many years of work-based practice. She has put in her 10,000 hours to become an expert. It then makes sense for visual artists to pair up with doctors in educating medical students for visual acumen, especially in the 'visual' specialties: radiology, dermatology and pathology (Bleakley et al. 2003a, 2003b). It surely makes a lot more sense to pair visual artists with, say, a dermatologist to take a group of medical students on a ward round to observe symptom patterns on the skin (with a briefing and debriefing educational opportunity with the dermatologist and artist in conversation with students about the differing ways that they 'look' and 'see') than to take the same group of medical students to an art gallery to learn how to look at pictures (Lesser 2018)?

The latter is commendable, but the former has immediate clinical benefit. Why not throw in a medical historian to debate the Levitican example discussed earlier and how this bears on what is seen in a contemporary dermatology clinic? Or involving an anthropologist would allow medical students to gain a cultural perspective on their work, perhaps frustrating potential medical imperialism (Bleakley et al. 2014). Rather than trek to the art gallery, scrutinised in more detail below (by the way, I have nothing against this – I am all for medical students looking at art; but there is also an art of looking to be learned in the clinic and on the wards), a better pedagogic proposal may be to set up regular life drawing classes shared with art students, a really good art tutor and an anatomist, for surface and living anatomy. This can be extended to sessions on reading scans and images with a radiologist and art historian. Not just as a 'throwaway' session but as core, integrated and assessed curriculum content. This way, medical students exercise the senses but also learn sensibility – aesthetic appreciation and judgement, and appreciation of, and wonder at, the body, rather than simply objectification and technical yield. While life drawing is now much more common for medical schools to offer (Price-Kuehne 2010), such classes are often not developed in terms of a 'maximum' educational opportunity (full complement of mixed professions tutors, plus imaginative pedagogy).

When the gallery becomes the ward

In 2011, my wife Sue, a visual artist, and myself ran a workshop at the Museum of Contemporary Art in Toronto (http://ago.ca/events/artists-diagnosticians-culture). We took 30 or so clinicians and medical educationalists on an art 'ward round'. The purpose was to take contemporary culture as the patient and use the available art to diagnose culture's ills, based on the ward round. We did not plan beforehand which pieces of art we would use, but allowed this to flow spontaneously from the round. Here, we followed Nietzsche's advice (expanded by Gilles Deleuze) that artists often act in the role of 'diagnosticians of culture' or 'symptomatologists' (Stivale 1998; Ahern 2010). As an example, we contemplated a collection of sculptural pieces by the Italian artist Guiseppe Penone (Basualdo 2018). Penone had carved out tree shapes horizontally from within recumbent trees, displaying an 'inner life'. This offers a radical shift from the usual mechanical visual trope of cutting a tree vertically to reveal its tree rings as a measure of annual growth. Penone shifts focus to the aesthetic of a tree birthing an inner tree. From the dead, cut tree perhaps a new tree springs, the outer tree representing the coffin.

Here we are at the bedside of Penone's sculpture. Let's leave the person – Penone himself and his motives and imagination – out of the conversation for the moment and let the sculptural object speak for itself. What symptoms does it show? What can we learn from close observation, or 'second looking'? The conversation then focused on the inner lives of trees and how trees might speak to us. This naturally led to talk about tree diseases and human intervention in the world of trees that is both destructive to the planet (mass deforestation) and instructive (forestry management). This in turn led to a discussion about the relationships between climate change, social inequality, social justice and global health. Close observation of Penone's sculptures also initiated talk of 'grain' – working with and against the grain; and of knots and 'crooked timber' or inherent flaws and paradoxes in the human condition.

Our perspective reversed the usual activity of public engagement – for example, taking people to galleries or museums, or the theatre – by focusing on the culture's symptoms rather than those of the individual (although these are clearly entangled). Chris Sharratt (2019), for example, describes 'Why Doctors Think Art Can Help Cure You', where "With art lessons and trips to museums on prescription, the links between culture and health are being reconsidered". This piece is published in *Frieze*, a leading visual art magazine, and not in a medical or medical education journal. Its audience is then the visual artist or curator, who is asked to be a diagnostician of culture, a symptomatologist. The article describes how the UK Government is launching a strategy to encourage doctors to engage patients with mild mental health issues in particular, such as depression and anxiety, in the arts – this, rather than prescribing antidepressants. Arts in health practitioners will tell you that this is a case of closing the stable door after the horse has bolted – such arts interventions have been practiced since at least the end of the Second World War and usually with little central funding help and often heaps of skepticism (Bates et al. 2013). Nevertheless, many hospitals have an artist-in-residence programme or support 'arts for health' activities.

Chris Sharratt's article describes a scheme in Montreal where patients are prescribed visits to the Montreal Museum of Fine Arts for a dose of culture, just as they might be prescribed exercise for obesity (Kelly 2018). But this is explicitly widening focus from mental to physical health issues. Brendan Kelly summarises such benefits from a number of studies, where engaging with art can increase levels of cortisol and serotonin, good for people with diabetes and other chronic illnesses. Of course, there is a glitch here. Who can tell what sort of art will have such positive health effects?

Will a Francis Bacon painting, a Chapman Brothers sculpture or a Marina Abramovic performance invite floods of cortisol and serotonin? Art does not necessarily set out to 'heal' or 'soothe', but usually to challenge, often upset, and certainly to make us 'think otherwise' and 'see otherwise'. And art often embraces political agendas of resistance against the mainstream. Art may take the very symptoms of society that it sets out to address and expand or indulge these symptoms, as parody, such as Jeff Koons' pop art, some of the most expensive and sought after pieces in the high-end market. Is this curative of culture or does it add another layer to symptom? Is a parody of consumerism that produces an elite consumer object a healthy option? Certainly it diagnoses some of the ills of culture, as noted above. Whatever the sociological implications, prior to that is the perceptual – we must look closely to arrive at a diagnosis.

But art too has a message for medicine in its cultivation of the 'original' and 'singular'. Famously, Andy Warhol took the phenomenon of mass production and subverted this by producing 'one off' mass produced items, such as screen prints, that have become collectors' pieces fetching obscene prices at auction. The point for medical practice is that mass production medicine – treating patients as numbers – should never compensate for the priceless one-off, singular experience of an excellent consultation.

In the examples above, we have taken the ward into the gallery, even though we have given this a twist by considering cultural symptoms rather than personal symptoms. Paradoxically, accounts of education of 'looking' and 'seeing' in medicine have concentrated on the flow from the hospital and clinic to the art gallery. This is another contradiction in medical education's attempt to educate for sensibility. Surely it makes more sense for visual artists to be brought in to the hospital and clinic, to input to ward rounds and consultations wherever patient consent can be obtained and confidentiality is not at risk? After all, clowns, musicians and social science researchers often input into hospital wards.

Honing visual acumen in medicine

Let us trace this – perhaps misguided – trajectory of two decades of research that has taken medical students and doctors out of the clinic and into the gallery to look at how visual sense may be educated or honed. In 2001, Ruric Anderson and colleagues (2001), from the Department of Medicine at the Medical College of Wisconsin, called for a rethink of how to teach visual close noticing in the physical examination, in an environment in which such skills were being slowly eroded. In the same year, Bardes and colleagues (2001) at Weil Cornell Medical College, New York, concerned about medical students' inability to read patients' emotional states through facial expressions, took students to an art gallery and taught them how to observe, describe and interpret portraits. A study at Yale University, also in 2001, studied whether systematic and coached 'looking' at figurative representational paintings could improve the observational skills of first year medical students with reference to skin conditions (Dolev et al. 2001). Students took pre- and post-test scores on what they noticed on standardised dermatology photographs. Eighty-one students then looked at paintings and discussed them, where 65 students made up a control group without the intervention. The coached group, however, showed only a 10% increase in positive recognition scores over the control group and there was no way of knowing if this small improvement lasted or decayed.

This first flush of research at the opening of the new millennium led Shapiro et al. (2006: 2623) to note that "medical educators have periodically experimented with using arts-based training to hone observational acuity". Well, at this point – 2006 – there were actually very few published accounts. The authors set out "to better understand the similarities and differences between arts-based and clinical teaching approaches to convey observation and pattern recognition skills". In a matched cohorts comparison of just 38 third year medical students, the authors found that tailored clinical activity to improve pattern recognition and hone observation did improve these abilities in this group of students. The clinical activity group benefitted most from learning about pattern recognition, possibly because of the relevance of the material. However, an arts-based approach added value, where "students also developed skills in emotional recognition, cultivation of empathy, identification of story and narrative, and awareness of multiple perspectives". Pitting the 'clinical' approach against the 'arts' approach is a hangover from the tired CP Snow 'Two Cultures' debate of arts/humanities versus science/technology, where a more productive approach is to twin the arts and sciences and to educate for clinical artistry.

At the Department of Family Medicine, University of Cincinnati, Nancy Elder and colleagues (2006) claimed that "teaching the skill of observation is often shortchanged in medical education". They set up an elective for 17 second year medical students through a medicine-art museum collaboration for teaching the 'Art of Observation'. An online evaluation suggested that the course had improved the students' clinical skills in observation and description. But how much authentic clinical work placement did these students actually experience? Again, why not bring the art museum expertise into the ward round, working with students at their coalfaces, amplifying their clinical observations through the input of the peripatetic artist?

At University College London medical school, Deborah Kirklin and colleagues (2007) systematically evaluated the effects of an arts-based educational intervention on the development of observational skills in primary care of both doctors and nurses. They focused on capability in diagnosing and referring suspicious pigmented skin lesions. The experimental group received an arts-based, 90 minutes long observational skill training (delivered by an artist), where the control group received practical training in the management of psoriasis. A significant difference in the quality of judgement between the two groups in favour of the arts-based intervention group was shown. The intervention was fairly simple – the artist gave participants common objects such as a coconut, a piece of carpet, some bubblewrap, an orange and a piece of broccoli to handle unseen, and then asked the participants to handle the same objects seen, describing tones, colours, shades and so forth in detail. All participants then described three photographs of dermatological symptoms. There was no longitudinal dimension to the study, so effects may not have lasted. But the main point here is that it was the artist who introduced new ways of looking closely at objects, expanding the perceptual registers and possibly capabilities, of the doctors and nurses.

Boudreau et al. (2008), at McGill University, Canada, simply asked an expert panel just what constitutes expert close noticing in medicine. They distilled four pedagogical principles and eight core principles of clinical observation as a basis to developing a course in clinical observation for first year medical students. The main educational principle is that learning must occur in live clinical contexts, challenging the dominant emerging paradigm of learning in museums and transferring to clinical contexts. The ward must become the gallery. Of the eight core principles, perhaps the most important is that "observation is distinct from inference" – students must describe what they see and not what they expect to see.

Naghshineh and colleagues' (2008) 'Training the Eye: Improving the Art of Physical Diagnosis' – a course in visual literacy – was offered for first and second year medical students at Harvard in 2004–05. Structured observation of artworks and a life drawing session were linked to patient care. Twenty-four students took the course and 34 were used as a control group. There was subsequently a significant difference between the two groups on reading clinical symptoms through photographs. A study such as this may be more meaningful if conducted with third and fourth year students who have greater clinical experience than years 1 and 2.

A study by Samy Azer (2011), based at the King Saud University College of Medicine in Saudi Arabia, showed that medical students learn surface anatomy of the abdomen more effectively through drawing rather than just verbally. Other studies – quoted in Azer (ibid) – have shown that students learn surface anatomy effectively through drawing on the skin. These visually oriented studies have a well-developed literature. This suggests that students should not simply be learning from artists and applying this to practice but should be doing art themselves, perhaps with artists facilitating rather than teaching. While arts-based observation education studies reported so far suggest benefits, they suffer from lack of hands-on experiential learning, craved by medical students.

Looking and seeing are, however, coloured by context. The largely functional approaches to examining close noticing could be extended to include affective influences upon the gaze in clinical practice. There is a difference between a physical examination performed on somebody who disgusts you as opposed to a patient for whom you feel warmth, attraction or respect, despite claims for professional neutrality. Further, the conditions under which physical examination is learned matters – for example, if the clinical teacher is supportive or resorts to poor pedagogical tactics such as ritual humiliation and pimping.

Elizabeth Gaufberg, a physician and educator, and Ray Williams, a director of education at a university art museum, developed 'The Personal Responses Tour' (Gaufberg and Williams 2011). Medical students are asked to think of a memorable patient – such as one you found it difficult to empathise with – and then find a work of art that somehow resonates with that patient, dwelling on and articulating the connections. The task is in-depth, taking one and a half hours. Here, art potentially plays a therapeutic/cathartic role. Who should facilitate such experiences however – an artist, a clinician or a psychologist or psychotherapist?

Catherine Belling (2011) points to the contradiction between what medical students and doctors actually feel and what she 'should' feel in exercising professionalism. Professionalism can be seen to demand discretion rather than confession. The widespread use of 'reflective practice' through narration can lead to medical students and doctors in pedagogical contexts 'faking it', deliberately avoiding self-disclosure in narratives. To recover authenticity, Belling notes that reflection as self-disclosure can occur through the medium of a "third thing" such as a painting. Here, a resonance is achieved through indirection.

At the University of Southern California Keck school of medicine, in collaboration with Los Angeles' Museum of Contemporary Art, Schaff et al. (2011) bucked the trend in medicine-art research and pedagogy projects for teaching observation using portraits or figurative art. Non-representational or abstract art might be just as important to study, as this carries a high level of ambiguity, and education for tolerance of ambiguity is key to medicine. Further, in observing, describing and interpreting non-representational artworks students engage in collaborative thinking and appreciation. A stepwise process is learned of collaborative close noticing, pattern recognition, matching to experience, engaging with multiple hypotheses and testing these, allowing intuitive judgement. This kind of collective appreciation and reasoning in the visual realm is familiar in say, multidisciplinary case meetings.

Michael Baum (McKie 2011), a surgical oncologist and Visiting Professor of Medical Humanities at University College, London, approaches paintings in a quite different way to extract literal forensic clues rather than to teach principles of looking. Painters learned from dissection but also from close study of the dead. A 15th-century painting – 'The Death of Procris' or 'A Satyr Mourning Over a Nymph' – by Piero di Cosimo in the National Gallery, London, shows a dead woman, a Nymph, mourned by a Satyr (www.nationalgallery. org.uk/paintings/piero-di-cosimo-a-satyr-mourning-over-a-nymph).

The setting suggests that the woman has been killed accidently by a spear during a deer hunt. Close examination of the painting, however, suggests Baum, shows that both hands "are covered with deep lacerations. There is only one way she could have got those. She has been trying to fend off an attacker who has come at her, slashing in a frenzied manner with a knife or possibly a sword". The woman's left hand is bent back in a way that suggests she has received a serious injury at points C3 and C4 on the cervical cord, causing nerve damage that would flex the fingers exactly as painted by di Cosimo.

A diagnostic 'ward round' in the gallery could continue in this way – for example, a self-portrait of Rembrandt shows that he was probably suffering from rosacea, reddening the facial tissues. This activity certainly links art and medicine in a fascinating way. But just what do students gain from diagnosing diseases in representational painting that they could not get from seeing patients on the ward or in a family practice with a visual artist in attendance scaffolding their 'learning to look', further extended for educational benefit through a briefing and debriefing?

Such forensics on Old Masters also seem somehow distanced from the contemporary world of the medical student and may seem arcane. Would students not equally enjoy and learn from study of Andres Serrano's large-scale photographs from the morgue (www.artnet.com/usernet/awc/awc_thumbnail.asp?aid=424202827&gid=424202827&cid=118026&works_of_art=1)? Or from the Scottish artist Christine Borland's re-personalisations of a woman's and a man's skulls used for anatomy teaching and bought directly from an osteological supplier? Here, helped by forensic scientists, Borland 're-fleshed' the bones as bronze heads to recover the persons – an Asian female and male (a 1966 piece called *Second Class Male, Second Class Female*) (Borland 2006). Borland was surprised, indeed shocked, to find that, at the time, she could buy a human skeleton from a catalogue used by anatomy departments in medical schools. This is no longer possible. This work serves as a metaphor for the need to educate for a personalising medicine rather than the dominant mode of de-personalising through objectifying patients.

More recently, Jaclyn Gurwin and colleagues (2018) at the University of Pennsylvania Perelman School of Medicine teamed up with educators at the Philadelphia Museum of Art to look at how 18 medical students' observational skills in the field of ophthalmology might be improved through art observation, description and interpretation. The results showed a significant improvement in observational recognition skills among those students who took the art observation course compared with a control group of 18 students.

The study claimed that just nine hours of art observation had a significant effect on observational skills. Such observation was purposefully active – including creative questioning, reasoning and perspective taking, reminding us that education of 'looking' is not a passive process, but involves cognitive and affective issues such as reflection and empathic engagement. Assessments included description testing and emotional recognition testing of retinal and facial disease photographs. While the study claims that a post-study questionnaire indicated that students who received the observational education had begun to apply the acquired skills usefully in "clinically meaningful ways", as first year medical students this must have been limited. And we are talking about a very small cohort, so again experimental design confounds results. What is important is the anatomy of the claimed learning: more accurate diagnostic close noticing in a visually complex clinical situation. Empathy and emotional recognition, such as noting affect in works of art, did not improve as a result of the intervention.

Gelgoot et al. (2018), in another North American study, conducted a review of the literature identifying medical education curricula that incorporate the visual arts. Only 15 articles met inclusion criteria. These studies claimed value for employing the visual arts to learn diagnostic acumen, communication and professionalism in particular. The authors note a dual purpose for education of visual acumen: first, diagnostic capabilities, and second, identifying with patients' experiences (educating for tolerance of ambiguity and the holding of multiple perspectives).

Neha Mukunda and colleagues (2019) also reviewed the literature on visual arts education in medical education with far more rigour and reach than Gelgoot and colleagues' study above. They noticed a bias in such studies towards preclinical medical students, thus negating a lot of the potential power of learning close noticing for diagnostic acumen where immediate application to clinical work is not possible. Further, from their review, it can be noted that a marketing strategy mindset is beginning to emerge for "validated pedagogies" such as "Visual Thinking Strategies" or "Artful Thinking" that can taint the aesthetic purposes of using the medical humanities with instrumental goals. One can feel that the medical humanities are ripe for packaging. They note:

> There is evidence that structured visual arts curricula can facilitate the development of clinical observational skills, although these studies are limited in that they have been single-institution reports, short term,

involved small numbers of students and often lacked controls. There is a paucity of rigorous published data demonstrating that medical student art education training promotes empathy, team building, communication skills, wellness and resilience, or cultural sensitivity.

The authors suggest that "more robust, evidence-based approaches for using visual arts instruction in the training of medical students" should be employed.

There is, then, an already rich and developing literature on teaching close observation to medical students, with certain models, particularly the medical school–art museum link, becoming dominant in the field. But there is a long way to go in developing more sophisticated research and in challenging two sticking points in particular – most research is done with first year students and projects are at the periphery of the main medicine curriculum. A literature review by Perry and colleagues (2011) found no evidence for significant and lasting effects on behaviour of arts-based interventions in medical schools, but this is probably because such interventions have not been well designed. We should not throw out the baby with the bathwater – linking clinical observation with arts-based 'seeing' is almost certainly sound, but experiments designed to test this have generally been poorly designed, flawed in conception and execution. Again, it makes little sense to examine arts-based interventions in first and second year medical students who have little clinical experience under their belts. A systematic programme of research is needed in which longitudinal interventions are made and evaluated.

Despite Perry and colleagues' review, programmes based on looking at artwork in galleries and museums and then applying this to medicine are now ubiquitous. Andrew Jacques and colleagues (2012) at Ohio State University College of Medicine have teamed up with Columbus Museum of Art to develop a two hours' long programme for medical students in which art is observed critically and collaboratively. A critical thinking strategy – 'Observe, Describe, Interpret, Prove (ODIP)' – is used, that can be transferred back, for example, to use on a ward round where close observation of patients is necessary. Richard Pretorius and colleagues (2005) have documented such a course at Buffalo University. From studying paintings, first year students learn how observation can help through sensitising to visual cues such as colour, shape and form. Jasani and Sacks (2012) at Robert Wood Johnson Medical School, New Jersey, claim that utilising visual art can enhance the clinical observational skills of medical students. But, although their sample was adequate (110 students), the intervention was short (three hours). The students were drawn from Year 3, however, and so had some clinical experience. They studied art images using Visual Thinking Strategies (VTS) and made diagnoses from photographs of patients. Pre- and post-test scores showed a difference in the kinds of language that students used to describe symptoms.

Where pre-test descriptions involved generic descriptive (non-specific) words such as 'normal' and 'healthy', post-test descriptors involved specific language such as "Her left arm is flexed at the shoulder and elbow with the hand clenched in a fist". Post-test language included reference to patients' emotional states and surroundings and included more speculative thinking. Thus, not only were close observations heightened, but also interpretation and reflection increased, enriching observations. The authors note that this was a one-off study and may not have lasting effects. However, here are some interesting findings about shifts in language use linked to visual acumen.

The studies catalogued above perhaps do not innovate in the curriculum with enough force or central presence, but remain peripheral and do not have curriculum re-conceptualisation impact. Simply training for close observation in medicine is not the same as, for example, challenging the nature of the structural, endemic masculine diagnostic gaze – this is the bigger project of democratising and feminising medicine. Further, does the 'art' itself matter? To artists, curators and art historians of course it matters. Yet the medical humanities culture blithely talks of using 'art' – particularly visual art – as if this were a generic category, without discrimination such as styles and quality. It is quite different to contemplate a grisly and challenging performance art piece involving, say, cutting or piercing the flesh than a representational painting such as Luke Fildes's 'The Doctor' – perhaps the most studied and discussed of medical representations beyond Vesalius' anatomical drawings.

Given the focus in this book on the issue of how we manage the abject and associated emotional responses in medical students' development, surely art focusing on the abject, such as radical performance pieces (e.g., ORLAN, Marina Abramovic, Martin O'Brien, Stelarc, Ron Athey, Kira O'Reilly and Gina Pane) may be more challenging and interesting for medical students to engage with than more staid representational painting. For example, in the Naghshineh and colleagues (2008) study above, students were asked to study Gauguin, Turner, Sargent, Munch, Picasso, Steen, Manet, Pollock and Monet mainly to look at abstract features such as pattern, colour, composition and form. Given that one of the criticisms of the use of art in medical humanities in medical education is that studies in museums may lack transfer to the bedside, would the same not apply to the art that is chosen here to represent principles? I have nothing against these artists, but what would be 'hot' for contemporary medical students may be to study contemporary performance artists as noted above, asking questions about the status of the body, particularly the medicalised body, including the gendered body, the human immunodeficiency virus (HIV) positive body, the dysmorphic body, self-harming, the drugged body, the body in pain and so forth. Martin O'Brien, for example, bases his art practice around living his cystic fibrosis and the shadow of its prognosis, performing the condition (O'Brien and MacDiarmid 2018).

Visual artists such as Christine Borland, mentioned above, ask questions about medicine's depersonalisation processes, focusing not on their own bodies but on how medicine treats bodies. Borland's (2006) body of work over more than two decades has consistently wrestled with issues that arise from the medical culture's view of the 'normal' body. Students may also relate more easily to a comix/graphic artist such as Ian Williams (2014, 2019), who is also a general practitioner. ORLAN (www.orlan.eu) does not deal with abstractions and principles of close noticing but with shaping the body through surgery to challenge gender stereotypes and to illustrate the 'theatre' or performative side of surgery. Ron Athey (www.ronathey.com) performs the body perceived as abject – the marginalised and stigmatised body. Ian Williams (www.graphicmedicine.com) confesses that your local GP is likely to be neurotic or carries symptoms but is not allowed to expose or explore these.

With the singular exception of Paul Macneill (2011), commentators have failed to inquire into why the arts employed generally in the medical humanities are "benign and servile in relation to medicine". As Macneill points out, treating the arts as a mere "resource" rather than a vehicle for critique is both missing an opportunity and demeaning. While all kinds of art may provide a 'third space' for 'thinking otherwise' about medical culture, clinical practice, identity construction and professionalism, not taking up the opportunity to draw on contemporary art focusing on medical themes in the medical humanities is surely to look a gift horse in the mouth.

Caroline Wellbery and Rebecca McAteer (2015) note that observational skills learned through medical education have been honed by a supplement of arts-based observation interventions in many medical schools – again usually visits to art galleries or museums where curators or art historians help students to notice more closely. Education of sensibility recovers what specialisation may have driven out – the ordinary perceptions in human encounters that allow for sensitivity to the Other. Wellberry and McAteer, both doctors, suggest that beyond education in arts-based observation, nature writing serves as a model for educating close observation. This may appeal to medical students as natural history overlaps so clearly with receiving a patient's history. Further, close reading of texts can encourage close reading of the patient as text, a point elaborated by Bleakley et al. (2011). Finally, medical students must be able to say what they see in terms of public narrative, and "the ability to craft this speech as public narrative" (Wellberry and McAteer 2015) is surely at the heart of a humane, patient-centred practice. Importantly, Wellberry and McAteer see the honing of sensibility as opening a door for resistance – where medical students and doctors can turn their newly honed gazes upon the institution of medicine itself, not just critically but constructively, in formulating appropriate interventions.

Usually, the focus of studies catalogued above is on developing, first, better observational capability and, second, interpretive capabilities; but also the power of the visual arts to elicit an emotional response in the observer is often recognised. Bringing these three components together is the goal of numerous contemporary art-and-medicine classes that, again, often take place in museums and may be led by museum educators, curators and art historians. For example, Florence Gelo at Drexel University College of Medicine describes how she brings doctors in a Family Medicine residency training programme to Philadelphia art museums and encourages them to describe to each other their emotional responses to a painting, to notice details and to interpret. (See annotation of "The HeART of Empathy: Using the Visual Arts in Medical Education" and its accompanying online video in the Literature, Arts, and Medicine Database, New York University – http://litmed.med.nyu.edu.)

In the following chapter, I look more closely at how we might research diagnostic visual work in medicine.

Note: Parts of this chapter and Chapter 7 appeared in an earlier and different form in Chapter 6, Alan Bleakley, *Medical Humanities and Medical Education: How the Medical Humanities Can Shape Better Doctors* (Routledge 2015). That work has been revised, updated and expanded to include new research.

7 Doing and researching aesthetic work in the visual domain

The eyes have it

One would think that ophthalmology education would engage with cutting edge ideas in visual studies, but this is not necessarily the case. An exception is described in Adam Baim's (2018) 'Getting the Picture: Visual Interpretation in Ophthalmology Residency Training'. Baim is an opthalmologist who, during residency training, carried out a six months' long ethnographic study of how eye doctors make clinical judgements. What Baim describes is both an explicit and tacit level to visual interpretation: "the disciplining of the trainee's attentions". Also, as part of an identity construction within the specialty, trainees follow "acculturation into expected styles of communicating visual interpretations to others". Visual education involves both values and dispositions and technical capabilities. The latter is a reasoning process naturally framed by the visual realm as both the subject of the specialty and the medium through which the specialty's diagnostic processes are realised. Turning 'looking' into 'seeing' is then an education of

i   Vigilant attention (see Chapter 2) or close attention to detail in a focused looking.
ii Paradoxical attention (see Chapter 2) or a 'floating attention' that is the embedding of the practitioner in the particular context of looking, or an awareness of ecological perception and whatever the environment affords. This is a tacit level to looking, where expertise kicks in as Type 1 reasoning or pattern recognition.
iii The shaping of an identity – the gaining of expertise turns into a connoisseurship as the opthalmologist becomes 'specialist'. This further involves full identification with the community of practice and its historical traditions, as a processional apprenticeship, while there is room for innovation to expand the specialty's knowledge and practice bases. Here, values guide ways of looking, as professional practice. Opthalmologists learn to be face-to-face intimate and practice touch (see Chapter 8), albeit highly localised. This can be uncomfortable for patients and requires the doctor also to be sensitive to the secondary meaning of

'how do I look?' by maintaining personal hygiene and managing impression management.

iv   A narrative sensibility. Opthalmologists, like all doctors, must be able to narrate symptoms to themselves, to patients and back to other doctors and health care practitioners in multi-disciplinary care and case meetings. The narrative will be embodied – utilising metaphors-in-the-flesh (Lakoff and Johnson 1980, 1999) to expand technical descriptions and give them greater presence and impact or to amplify meanings – and must translate technical language into lay language for patients' understandings and insights. Baim (2018: 816) encourages trainee opthalmologists to collaboratively 'speak aloud' their diagnostic observations to form a narrative that coalesces into a diagnosis or differential diagnosis. This implies a particular pedagogy, where "Further research is needed to characterise how the performance of speech genres shapes the interpretive skills of medical trainees" (ibid). Baim then suggests that the close looking required of opthalmologists can be taken as an overall close scrutiny that should run through their bodily and verbal practices – close attention, talk and adherence to a logic of diagnosis. The vision of the opthalmologist's practice itself should not be blurred or occluded.

Opthalmologists have deepened their understanding of their own discipline reflexively by widening study of the eye out from the medico-biological to the literary, where the eye acts as a metaphor ('all-seeing', 'an instrument of surveillance', 'seat of the soul' and so forth) (Amm 2000). Panayotov (2017), drawing on Mesopotamian medical texts largely from the first millennium BCE, notes the breadth and richness of metaphors relating to eye symptoms and underlying diseases such as blood deposits, colour, atypical movements, sores and foreign objects in the eye. These provided an embodied language not only for enriching clinical understanding of eye conditions but also for teaching purposes and for enlivening conversation with patients.

Other medical and surgical specialties have devised pedagogical techniques based around education of vision. For example, Mina Arsanious and Gavin Brown (2018) describe teaching electrocardiogram interpretation through linking looking to drawing, so that more than one sense is fully engaged. Cope and colleagues (2015) describe how to both teach and learn the interpretation of visual cues during surgery. The authors note that surgeons may show confidence in motor skills while lacking expertise in attending to visual cues, creating a mismatch. Further, education in making judgements in the visual realm is neglected in surgical education.

Cope and colleagues' study developed an innovative research design drawing on multiple methods: case study (12 postgraduate surgical trainees), video and audio recordings and observer field notes – combined to gain profiles of teacher–trainee interactions with over 11 hours of observations. Analysis involved drawing out major themes from the data through constant comparison. Visual cue interpretation was found to be a central feature of teacher–trainee interactions, described by the research as 'co-constructed' or 'dialogical'. The eye is educated not just by looking but also by multiple sensory attention, including specialist embodied language. Importantly, co-construction involved not only confirmation of known anatomy, physiology and pathology but also co-construction of tolerance of ambiguity where neither teacher nor trainee was sure of what was being observed, but could form a working hypothesis. Trainees did not see naively but were taught to see, and this involved triadic alignment of activity that turned 'looking' into 'seeing': visual observation, augmented visual observation through laparoscopic instruments, and embodied language interventions and exchanges (verbal and non-verbal).

Making sense of diagnosis

Consider this description of a nurse at work:

> Around midnight he started getting a bit more pale ... and his lung sounds were ok. They had a few crackles but nothing really significant ... by about 2am he was looking quite a bit worse and very wet ... So I got blood gas and the pH was 7.2 ... I finished giving the bicarb about a half hour previously and I looked at the baby and he looked much worse than he had before ... His mouth was just open slightly. He was gasping to try to breathe. He just looked awful, looked absolutely terrible ... So I gave the Lasix (*Furosemide*, a diuretic), but at that point the baby was looking so bad that I didn't even wait for the Lasix to take effect before I went ahead and did another blood gas.
>
> (Benner et al. 2009: 117)

Albeit rather dated, this account beautifully illustrates the ocular-perceptual basis (and bias, in an ocular-centric culture) to health care. The decisions made to treat this ill baby were grounded in a close noticing of qualities, primarily visual ("getting a bit more pale", "looking quite a bit worse"); but auditory cues are also involved – "lung sounds" as "crackles". Sensitivity too is involved ("He just looked awful, looked absolutely terrible"). Ways of 'looking', embedded within a moral practice of concern and care, are central to diagnostic acumen and, again, may be best educated through clinicians working in tandem with those whose primary work is also 'looking', such as visual artists and art historians. The latter, of course, 'care' mainly for material objects. It is their aesthetic concern that underpins beautiful architecture, elegant instruments, engaging film and television and so forth, again as 'diagnosticians of culture' in Nietzsche's phrase (Ahern 2010). My point is that morality informs an aesthetic. Sensitivity encompasses ethical care, where sensibility is *aesthetic labour*, such as the expressive close noticing of the nurse in the example above. Medical aesthetics complements the established field of medical ethics.

Let us return to the nurse above, making qualitative judgements based on sense impressions, or doing aesthetic work. In 1859, Florence Nightingale (in Quain 1883: 1038) wrote that close noticing is "The *sine qua non* of being a nurse", where "attending to ... one's own senses ... should tell the nurse how the patient is". This is the aesthetic labour of health care. Again, who would wish for an an-aesthetic or insensible health care service? This would be dull, uninspired, ugly, unimaginative, flat, clumsy, insensitive, tiresome and numbing. Aesthetic work is elegant, inspiring, beautiful, imaginative, animated, dignified, graceful, sensitive, distinctive and passionate. In the context of art history, Rudolf Arnheim (1969: 206) describes a sophisticated kind of looking as "intelligent vision", but reminds us that this "cannot be confined to the art studio". Arnheim suggests that such intelligent vision can succeed in other disciplines "only if the visual sense is not blunted". We must, in Arnheim's phrase, "think with the senses" and think acutely. As the art historian James Elkins (2003: preface) suggests: "Most sciences have specific visual competencies and these present 'ways of seeing' waiting to be explored".

Nearly a half century ago, the philosophers of science Michael Polanyi and Harry Prosch (1975: 31) argued that education of the senses is essential for good science, where

> no science can predict observed facts except by relying with confidence upon an art: the art of establishing by the trained delicacy of eye, ear, and touch a correspondence between the explicit predictions of science and the actual experience of our senses to which these predictions shall apply.

Bardes et al. (2001: 1157) noted that "clinical diagnosis involves the observation, description, and interpretation of visual information", where such skills "are also the special province of the visual arts". The arts, it seems, offer essential capital for distribution across to the culture of medicine in educating for close noticing. But does this work? Chapter 6 discussed what evidence from studies tells us, but we saw that such studies are generally poorly designed leading to ambiguous results and are often framed in terms of confrontation between art and science, rather than the benefits of mutuality as interdisciplinary conversation. The common focus of such limited studies is education of visual observation in museums and galleries that may then be transferred to clinical contexts. This approach is interesting, often valuable, but flawed. Again, why not study looking and seeing in contexts of work (doctors in clinical worlds, artists in their studios) and set up conversations between them to see what this yields? This draws us away from seeking 'proof' in the value of educational interventions to seeking meaning and understanding.

In the previous chapter, I also gave an account of how my wife Sue and I purposefully subverted these museum-based studies by turning a tour around an exhibit in Toronto into a 'ward round' in which the 'patients' were the artefacts, the art pieces themselves. The art came to act as media and metaphors for ways in which diagnostic decisions are made in the visual realm. The artefacts, just like diagnostic technologies, come to expand not just our sensing but also our learning, that becomes 'expansive' (Engeström 2019). The danger comes where the artefact fails to network with the person who is using it, so that it becomes a 'runaway' or 'wildfire' object – now superseding human sense. This produces the paradox of a senseless instrument.

Artists and doctors collaborate in 'thinking aloud'

Alan Bleakley and colleagues (Bleakley 2004; Bleakley et al. 2003a, 2003b) describe an award-winning (*Journal of Workplace Learning* paper of the year) research project on 'ways of seeing' that attempted to anatomise and theorise sense perception within the domain of medical expertise, where visual artists and doctors were paired in 'thinking aloud' conversations. The method involved analysis of videotaped conversations between artists and physicians about profession-specific ways of looking and seeing, where artists visited clinics and physicians visited artists' studios.

One element that emerged from this research was how expertise may either reach a comfortable plateau that becomes habitual, or may continue to develop as a generative connoisseurship. This challenges the often blithely accepted 10,000 hours rule of expertise first introduced by Malcolm Gladwell (2008) in *Outliers: The Story of Success*. While practice does obviously increase expertise, it may not lead to connoisseurship but may plateau at levels of adequate competence rather than outstanding capability (hungry for more and innovating).

In the study in question, experienced physicians said that comparing their work with that of experienced artists had challenged their comfort zones and rekindled their passion in the artistry of visual diagnosis. In Japanese, a distinction is made between 'ordinary seeing' and 'active seeing'. In English, this is equivalent to the distinction between mere 'looking' and active 'seeing'. 'Active seeing' in Japanese is used, for example, to describe a doctor looking at a patient. The same word (*miru*) also means 'to have sexual relations' and a 'stolen look'. This deeper kind of seeing is then eroticised – *passionate*, or life giving. Experts said that although they had developed considerable skill in close noticing, this often felt less than passionate and talking with artists has re-kindled the desire to 'look again' with a fresh eye.

Can doctors then benefit from collaboration with artists in inquiry into clinical judgement practices and will this lead to a new identity construction? Bleakley and colleagues' methodology draws on traditions of collaborative action research, participative inquiry (Reason 1994) and appreciative inquiry (Cooperrider and Whitney 1999). Appreciative inquiry emphasises that while practice may already be good, continuous reflection, as an art in itself, can bring further enhancements. This approach also stresses passionate, heart-felt involvement with subject matter, rather than cool detachment, as a legitimate research stance. The methodology is grounded in identity constructions through resistance to regulative and normative discourses, following the trajectory of Michel Foucault's late work (Bernauer and Rasmussen 1994) where processes of 'aesthetic self-forming' are described as patterns of resistance to culturally-determined norms of self-presentation, the latter also a form of surveillance and control. In Chapter 9, I consider the issue of such surveillance and control in medical students' and doctors' self-presentation in terms, for example, of dress codes, giving 'how do I look?' a double meaning. Again, education of the senses in medicine is intimately bound with identity constructions and is as much a political and ethical issue as an aesthetic one.

The dominant discourse of technical medical judgement marginalises aesthetic approaches to practice and constructs doctors as technicians. It also neatly bypasses political or power interests – for example, where the education of insensibility in medical students is challenged, or where a redistribution of sensibility capital is called for. I have experienced this many times in teaching medical students, where unfounded assumptions about the emotional maturity of a young medical student is challenged, thus redistributing emotional labour capital; or where a method of teaching and learning is inappropriately used (dulling the senses of the students) and is properly challenged and adapted.

Where artists are familiar with forming images, medical students and doctors may form aesthetic and ethical identities through appreciation of clinical images, as a basis to expertise in a specialty. The ethical part is where such images (a) show pathology and (b) have sources in persons. An ethically appropriate approach to this presentation is to respect the patient and his or her suffering through acknowledgement. In the project described below, the artists' interventions have focused the doctors on the inherent aesthetic of the "informational" images (Elkins 1999) they habitually meet with an objectifying medical gaze (tacitly avoiding acknowledgement of either suffering or personhood of the patient). The artists also model the value of generation, rather than reduction, of uncertainty.

The project was unusual in its interest in identity formation as a research outcome and added another twist to this approach where it shifted the focus of the doctor's identity away from personality towards how the doctor gives respectful metaphorical personality to the presenting clinical image as if this were an art piece. Typically, a specialty such as pathology strives to reduce uncertainty at all costs, but in the process may lose the tolerance for ambiguity that is the hallmark of deliberate practice (Fish and Coles 1998). Where clinical judgement is restricted to, and by, technical procedure and protocol, and then loses its "artistry" (Schön 1990), we can characterise this as being authoritarian towards the image. Less reflective 'image authoritarians' may be more prone to classic diagnostic errors, such as premature closure, by not seeking alternative or innovative explanations (Schmidt and Boshuizen 1993).

Research data were gathered in a number of ways and in differing forums:

- Public seminar and debate, and conference presentations: these formal settings, documented through videotaping, audiotaping and notes, involved framing of typical episodes of clinical and aesthetic judgements in the visual domain, to which invited audiences of doctors and artists responded.
- 'Thinking aloud' work-based exchanges (artists to clinics and doctors to studios). These allowed practitioners to swap live practices and stories. The deliberative and reflective processes were documented through extensive notes.
- Doctors talking to clinical images such as X-rays, pathology slides and photographs of skin conditions. These model typical clinical formulation responses and were audiotaped and transcribed.
- Minuted review and round table discussions progressing models and insights with the project convenor, a medical educator and psychologist. This was an iterative process.

Data were triangulated with a literature review and expert opinion culled from presentations within the local medical and medical education community. Data analysis followed grounded theory principles in coding, categorising and model building. In summary, five kinds of practice were noted:

1 *Habitual practice.* Experts may see what they habitually expect to see and not notice what is there, so that 'perceptual readiness' occludes fresh seeing. This calls for an outside challenge to 'describe what you see, not what you expect to see'. Here, 'seeing' is in a sense strictly policed within protocols and guidelines within a specialty, and within a local, processional tradition ('this is the way we do things around here'). Medical students and juniors are expected to conform to what seniors have acquired as habitual practices, to properly inhabit the 'habitus' of the community of practice (Bourdieu 1977). Habitual practice is then also a political practice, and exercise of sovereign power in framing what is legitimate.

2 *Saturated practice.* The expert eye may become tired through over exposure to everyday material and needs to be refreshed. This is linked with (1) above and calls for an outside challenge to reframe the conventions of 'looking', 'seeing' and 'saying' within the specialty. Doctors may need to be reintroduced to the conventions of their images as a re-framing through the interventions of visual artists.

3 *Restricted practice.* Experts may fail to gain a balance between an evidence-based, technical approach and idiosyncratic practice artistry.

The latter allows for greater tolerance of ambiguity and for innovation. It promotes a more flexible diagnostic capability under conditions of complexity, uncertainty, ambiguity, uniqueness and ethical conflict. Practitioners who employ such artistry tend to be interested in the value of heuristics as well as scientific objectivity, but are also more likely to collaborate with others in reaching judgements.

4   *Aesthetic practice.* This is a logical extension of (3) above and calls for an explicit acceptance that the work of diagnosis needs an educated sensibility of discrimination between qualities. This is an aesthetic, not a technical, dimension, although it is informed by technical (scientific) knowledge. Key here again is the forming of an aesthetic identity as a 'connoisseur'. Second, where such connoisseurship is of informational images, the aesthetic dimension can be extended to such images, so that the traditional distinction between informational, non-expressive or non-art, images and 'art' images is collapsed. Third, experts judiciously draw on a range of visual heuristics that offer vivid similitudes and metaphors, referring the clinical image back to a natural referent (Bleakley 2018). This tacit storehouse of images and metaphors prepares and enhances perception and then diagnostic acumen. Such a focus is characteristically avoided in traditional continuing education in the medical specialties.

5   *Ethical practice.* This is a logical extension of (4) above. Sensitivity to isolated matter of the body (an X-ray image, a pathology specimen, a photograph of a skin condition) is extended as a humanising move to embed that abstracted clinical interest and judgement back into the lives (and deaths) of patients. Such active movement between isolated sign, symptom and bodily matter or image and the phenomenological realities of patients is an active component in the forming of a doctor's identity as an ethical practitioner. This would offer a challenge to the traditional diagnostic gaze that dehumanises or objectifies.

Democratising the medical gaze in medicine

Close noticing, as argued above, is not simply naïve looking, but is a historically, culturally and socially formed process that can be conceived as capital, owned by experts and distributed by them according to structural rules of power. Aesthetics and politics – or sensibility, power and resistance – are intimately linked (Rancière 2006). The diagnostic looking, or 'gaze', of the doctor, has been widely studied and debated since its description by Michel Foucault (1991) as a surveillance gaze of power or authority as well as a scientific, objectifying gaze. Bleakley et al. (2011) and Bleakley (2014) argue that the democratisation of the medical gaze – as a form of educational resistance – through the rise of inter-professional teamwork and patient-centred practices serves to distribute the capital of the gaze amongst a wider group of stakeholders.

Further, the basis upon which the medical gaze is traditionally learned, that of dissection (see Chapter 2), is obviously dissolved in medical schools that do not include dissection as part of the process of learning anatomy (McLachlan and de Bere 2004; McLachlan et al. 2004). But the argument concerning distribution of the medical gaze has not yet entered this debate that is still centred mainly on functional availability of cadavers rather than a more sophisticated pedagogical debate about what is the best way to learn anatomy (Regan de Bere and Mattick 2010; Mushaiqri 2015), rather than the most effective initiation rite for medical students, or how to bring those students into intimate contact with death (Bishop 2011).

The work of Bleakley and colleagues described above explicitly sets out to challenge the dominance of the medical gaze through democratisation, by introducing an equal debating voice – that of the artist. The medical gaze or 'perception', the key performance element described in Foucault's (1976) account of the birth of the clinic (modern diagnostic medicine in the teaching hospital), rests on an idiosyncratic, socialised connection between 'seeing' and 'saying'. The act of looking deep into bodies through literal dissection is linked with an exclusive diagnostic vocabulary that affords an imperialism of the gaze. What the doctor says is 'true' (knowledge is power) and this is reinforced by it being said in the doctor's exclusive professional domain, the clinic (authority), to reinforce identities (that of the doctor and that of the patient). The 'gaze' is then not confined to literal sense-based diagnosis, but offers a metaphor for professional solidarity, making sense of medicine as a cultural discourse. While Foucault's use of the word 'gaze' is not restricted to the ocular, the eye is certainly privileged, reinforcing the wider ocular-centricity of western culture.

The direct gaze (vigilant attention) is explicitly taught in medical education, but the free-floating 'glance' (paradoxical attention) that Foucault briefly describes as a component of medicine's authority is picked up through socialisation into medical culture as an 'absorbed' aspect of habitus. The layperson is familiar with the glance as habitual 'thick looking' hovering between consciousness and the unconscious. It is active as an 'indwelling' of the world. The glance is also a central aspect of manners in Chinese culture, where direct eye contact is avoided as one 'glances off' another's glance as a mark of respect. The glance in medicine and medical education is virgin territory, wholly unexplored in associated research or theory as far as I know, although the phenomenologist Edward Casey (2007) has devoted a 500-page book to the topic. It is important in resisting the Western imperialism of medical education, where the direct gaze, as eye contact, is privileged in both medical practice and pedagogy (such as small group problem-based learning). In a number of cultures, including Asian and Native North American, direct eye contact is considered rude, where the glance is encouraged.

Within art history, Martin Jay (1993) mentions how the penetrating and direct gaze evolved from the glance. In the medical consultation, the glance and the gaze would serve differing purposes. The gaze fixes and controls in a monological fashion, where the glance is dialogical, indicating the doctor's continuing interest and presence without interrupting the patient. The characteristic medical gaze maintains sensibility capital for the doctor, where the glance affords distribution of such emotional labour capital.

Sensibility capital in medicine is a complex web of forces and not simple a repository of knowledge and skills. At the heart of this web is the identity construction of the doctor as specialist, whose connoisseurship can be perceived by laypersons as magical. This, of course, can inflate doctors' importance – the focus of a raft of anthropological and literary studies. For a recent confessional account of how one famous neurosurgeon has wrestled with the issue of self-importance, see Henry Marsh's (2014) *Do No Harm: Stories of Life, Death and Brain Surgery.*

Aesthetic ways of knowing in health care

Looking is part of the sensory or aesthetic ways of knowing central to every health care practice. Every clinical educationalist is surely familiar with the groundbreaking work of Donald Schön (1991) on the 'artistry' of professional practice, but few will have read the important work of Barbara Carper (1978) on aesthetic knowing in nursing. While both authors situate pedagogy primarily in aesthetics rather than in instrumental values, neither of these approaches has been formally progressed for references to aesthetic concerns. Donald Schön's work in particular has often been reduced to frames for instrumental skills acquisition or functional use of educational technologies. An exception to this is the work of Della Fish and Colin Coles (Fish and Coles 1998) on progressing Schön's view of practical knowing (itself derived from the pragmatism of John Dewey). They translate professional 'artistry' as "deliberative critical appreciation" of one's own practice, but explicitly ground this in ethics (moral inquiry) rather than aesthetics.

Schön's (1991) work on the development of judgement in the professions through reflective practice resulted in a description of the 'artistry' of professional practice. But Schön did not progress this idea through grounding in formal work on aesthetics (Bleakley 1999). Subsequent work on reflective practice as personal or procedural knowing in health care (Kember 2001; Freshwater and Jons 2005), while referring to both Schön's notion of 'artistry' and Carper's aesthetic way of knowing, has also not formally progressed the idea of practice artistry through grounding in aesthetic theory drawn from philosophy, cultural studies, art history and psychology. For example, work on visual intelligence and the visual mind shows a healthy interdisciplinary collaboration between scientists, social scientists, artists and art historians (Arnheim 1969; Jones and Galison 1998; Elkins 2003), but has hardly touched clinical education.

In a nursing education context, Carper (1978: 23) describes four "fundamental patterns of knowing" informing health care practice: empirics or scientific knowledge, personal or self-knowledge, ethics or moral knowledge and aesthetics, which she refers to as 'the art' of nursing. Carper refers to "the esthetic (sic) perception of significant human experiences", appropriately formulating aesthetics as the integration of sense impressions and acts of appreciation. However, while the four ways must overlap in practice, Carper separates ethics, or moral knowing, from aesthetics, where moral knowing is "the capacity to make choices within concrete situations involving particular moral judgements". Moral judgement can, however, be grounded in aesthetic appreciation or the development of a sensibility, where discrimination between qualities, close noticing and perceptual engagement with an Other precedes and forms the ethical act. This synthesis results in an aesthetic and ethical self-forming, or an identity construction as a sensitive and appreciative practitioner and a connoisseur of clinical symptoms (Bleakley 2004).

As both historical (Panayotov 2017) and cognitive psychology research (Lakoff and Johnson 1980, 1999; Bleakley 2018) indicate, the most complex expert decisions are grounded in thinking in metaphors, as schemata or coding constituting tacit knowing. In clinical reasoning in medicine, pattern recognition of a complex of symptoms can be explained as a match between the presenting patient and an 'illness script' that is a sophisticated encapsulation of knowledge as a network of metaphors and resemblances (Boshuizen and Schmidt 1995), discussed in Chapter 6. Expert judgement is often referred to as 'intuitive' or based on 'gut feeling', descriptors which tend to make the process mysterious rather than transparent. Advances in cognitive psychology that model representations of knowledge serve, however, to partly demystify expert knowing.

Arthur Reber's (1993) rigorous experimental psychology research demonstrates how people learn and store rules that they do not comprehend explicitly, but which help them to more expertly perform linguistic acts. People learn tacit transformational rules that they cannot explain but can nevertheless mobilise. Reber calls such learning "implicit", the storage of knowledge "tacit" and the site of storage "the cognitive unconscious". Resemblances or striking likenesses provide one important dimension to the architecture of a cognitive unconscious or tacit knowing. Many of these are visual, extending Reber's account beyond spoken language to visual language. Reber's "cognitive" unconscious, framing and informing Type 1 reasoning or pattern recognition, must extend to affect and performativity.

Resemblances

In medicine, there is a large vocabulary of resemblances that can act as heuristics or short cuts to diagnosis (Bleakley 2018). A 'strawberry gallbladder' (where the gallbladder has excess fat) uncannily resembles a ripe strawberry; a 'nutmeg liver' (where the liver is engorged with blood) resembles a cut nutmeg; an 'apple core lesion' on an X-ray showing colonic carcinoma shows a characteristic apple core shape and so forth. Experts do not like to encourage novices to resort to heuristics, preferring them to develop an analytical, differential diagnostic method in the absence of clinical experience. Experts themselves, however, regularly rely on pattern recognition as a short cut. Recall Abraham Verghese's (1999: 299) simultaneous warning and confession: "I taught students to avoid the 'blink-of-an-eye' diagnosis ... the snap judgement. But secretly, I trusted my primitive brain, trusted the animal snout".

Of course, heuristics bring the danger of bias, and this is well documented for the professions in general (Kahneman et al. 1982) and nursing in particular (Thompson and Dowding 2002; Palmer 2003). Fonteyn and Fisher (1995) argue that heuristics are particularly important in nursing judgements – that they characterise as less focused upon "diagnosis and hypothesis generation" and more upon the abilities to "distinguish between relevant and irrelevant patient data ... and to make decisions that assist in accomplishing the overall treatment plan for each patient". But this description does not address the rapidly changing face of nursing where Thompson and Dowding's (2002) prediction that "Nurses will increasingly be asked to diagnose disease" has come to fruition.

Indeed, it does not account for the host of everyday unspoken sense-based judgements that nurses make about patients that have stronger or weaker diagnostic consequences. Emphasising the potential biases and errors arising from the use of heuristics may be over-stated, or overshadowed by the larger spectre of the need to conform to evidence-based approaches. Shielding novices from engaging with pattern recognition early in their careers may deny the development of sense-based judgement acumen and certainly its acceleration or 'hothousing', for there is a further element to abductive reasoning that must now be discussed that is desirable to learn early in a health care career.

There is a final part to this puzzle of turning how we 'look' (surface looking) into how we 'see' diagnostically (deeper perception). We must be engaged with the patient, passionate about the work. 'Empathy', a weak and overused term word, does not capture such passion (Marshall and Bleakley 2017). Rather, we must think about the 'charge' of a health care relationship that is necessarily skin-to-skin (see Chapter 8), sometimes electric – even erotic, sometimes arousing disgust and often neutralised by a professional insensibility.

If we take the 'erotic' as an embodied metaphor rather than literally, the process of diagnostic seeing can be imagined as eroticised or given extra intensity and sensuality, while charged with compassion. As mentioned previously, in Japanese, a distinction is made between 'ordinary seeing' and 'active seeing' (Elkins 1999). 'Active seeing' (*miru*) is used to describe a doctor looking at a patient. Where the same word (*miru*) also means 'to have sex', we need not take this literally. Such deeper, eroticised 'seeing' (or engagement) is passionate or life giving. This reveals an ethical layer to the model of abductive reasoning developed here. The prior technical and aesthetic elements of a diagnostic judgement may be in place, but this is completed within an overall act of care that is the ethical gesture.

The visual rhetoric of clinical practice

This, and the previous, chapter argue for a formal education of what Florence Nightingale described as the "power of attending ... to one's own senses" in clinical judgement. Establishing a formal aesthetics of practice in a curriculum requires advice from experts in the field of aesthetics inviting medical humanities interventions in the medicine curriculum. However, the field of health care practice research can do much to help itself in developing a poetics of practice. First, as described earlier, it can formally build on the leads provided by Schön's notion of practice 'artistry' and Carper's aesthetic way of knowing. We can resist reducing artistry to functional (efficient cause) effects such as the 'training' of communication 'skills'. This merely leads us back to the technical rational 'high ground' that Schön suggests is not the best place from which to approach uncertainty, ambiguity, uniqueness and value conflicts in practice. Given that important instances of clinical judgement cannot simply be approached by technical-rational means, it is important to keep alive the study of heuristics and sense-based judgement in clinical reasoning. However, in an age of evidence-based health care, such forms of judgement are not developed well in the literature in comparison with technical-rational approaches such as decision analysis.

At the same time as we attempt to reduce uncertainty through fine discrimination, can we not also educate for tolerance of ambiguity? Here, we do not slip away from the diagnostic problem at hand to invoke technical-rational decision analysis modes too early in the process of judgement. In other words, can we save the art of bedside clinical judgement from the potentially suffocating grip of analytical decision models? The hope is to preserve close, imaginative and committed care of the patient, where compassion and sense-based judgement are two sides of the same coin. This is not to devalue the worth of decision analysis methods. Rather, again it is a plea to not lose the art of clinical judgement to such methods.

An aesthetic health care is sensitive, elegant and appreciative and faces up to the sublime, the terror of illness. It is, however, perhaps easier to grasp an aesthetic health care by what it is not: an-anaesthetic. To anaesthetise is to dull. We do not want our medical-educational practices to dull or be dulling, to be habitual, or to recycle tired conventions, re-iterated throughout this book. While we have developed a sophisticated health care pragmatics and ethics, the aesthetic arena has been neglected. This book calls for the urgent development of a sub-discipline of medical/health care aesthetics with the medical/health humanities as inspiration and source for curriculum development.

Kinds of reasoning in the senses

Following Aristotle, Martha Nussbaum (2001: 290) notes that medicine is a 'stochastic' art – that is, an art with a high degree of uncertainty and random chance. Novices in medicine suffer greatly from such randomness because they have not yet learned how to focus on salient features of a situation that give a greater sense of certainty – for example, learning how to recognise signs and symptoms in order to arrive at a diagnosis. But will such inherent uncertainty be eradicated by technologies? Where "technology has given us an extended eye" (Ursitti 2008: 2), is this merely extending the clinical gaze, or further objectifying patients, as 'hands-on' medicine becomes a distant memory? In classical bedside medicine, the eye rules supreme. In Abraham Verghese's 2009/2010 novel *Cutting for Stone,* the reader is asked to "See how her (the patient's) eyes keep roving as if she's waiting for something? A grave sign. And look at the way she picks at the bedclothes – that's called carphology, and those little muscle twitches are *subsultus tendinum*" – symptoms of typhoid fever.

To recap: as they gain expertise such as turning mere looking into diagnostic seeing, medical students come to form cognitive schemata – generalised representations formed from exposures to individual symptom types – that allow them eventually to make clinical judgements according to pattern recognition ('I know this, I've seen many before'). The opthalmologist and eye surgeon Haidar Al-Hakim (undated) www.thethirdeyedoctor. co.uk/why-the-third-eye/) calls this the development of a 'third eye'. Not an occult reference, but a metaphor for the development of a synthetic cognitive process that both shapes and makes sense of visual cues. But we have seen how we must widen from the 'cognitive' in clinical judgement to include the affective and performative. Pattern recognition, or non-analytical reasoning, becomes a form of 'tacit knowledge' or an 'indwelling' of a phenomenon (Polanyi 1983; Engel 2008). This kind of reasoning is again Type 1 or System 1, as opposed to rational, logical and deductive forms of reasoning following rules, as Type 2 or System 2. It is widely accepted that in everyday cognition, as well as in expert judgements, both forms of reasoning work together as a dual system (Frankish 2010).

Studies of eye tracking by doctors using visual skills during diagnostic process also show two processes at work – global impression and focal search. These can be compared to, respectively, paradoxical and vigilant attention, introduced in Chapter 2 and a recurring theme of this book. Where novices and juniors use mainly focal search, experts rely more on a global impression, a holistic grasp of the image. Global impression is like System 1 (holistic and intuitive) clinical reasoning, where focal search is like System 2 (logical, analytical) reasoning (Norman 2007). We might then 'hothouse' or accelerate the clinical reasoning capacities of novices through introducing deliberate, planned exposure to common visual stimuli – in other words, meet plenty of patients early in a medical education with emphasis upon expert guidance (scaffolding learning) through briefing and debriefing. This is enriched by 'learning how to see' through the medical humanities as core and integrated curriculum provision – perhaps a learning how to 'see otherwise'.

As William Osler said:

> Medicine is learned by the bedside and not in the classroom. Let not your conceptions of disease come from words heard in the lecture room or read from the book. See, and then reason and compare and control. *But see first.*
>
> (my emphasis)

To help medical students to progress 'looking' to 'seeing' needs expert seniors' guidance in clinical settings, but we can supplement and enrich this process by adding the gifts of visual arts and the expertise of visual artists to the mix.

8   Touch/don't touch

Of all the senses, touch perhaps carries the greatest ambiguity. We crave touch, touch is healing, comforting and denotes intimacy; at the same time, touch can be unwanted, uninvited, inappropriate or used as a controlling gesture. Touch can be gentle and caressing or used to restrain, cajole and bully. Touch can be a lifeline or a fuse, lighting a blue touchpaper as prelude to an explosion. In medicine, touch has a special place with dual signification – first, the instrumental touch of the physical examination and the intimate examination given non-intimately; second, appropriate intimate touch as a gesture of support and care. The secret of touch in medicine is surely to bring these two strands together, where the instrumental is suffused with compassion and artistry so that technique becomes a gesture of embrace.

Rusting at the bedside: medicine running out of touch

While touch is fundamental to the professional work of doctors and surgeons, it is relatively neglected in both practical and academic medical education as a formal topic of study (Kelly et al. 2014, 2018, 2019). Qualities and registers of touch, such as those embodied in traditional percussion as a diagnostic method, are disappearing facets of medicine. And yet touch embodies much more than just 'hands on' examination.

Martina Kelly, an Irish family practitioner now practicing in Calgary, has long advocated the value of touch in medical education and the need to articulate its qualities and to understand touch philosophically, drawing particularly on phenomenology to make sense of clinical work (Gillespie et al. 2018). What does it mean to touch, be touched and be in, or out of, touch? In the recovery of philosophies of embodiment after Descartes had relegated the body as secondary to the mind, phenomenology brings us back into touch with touch. A fourth year medical student that I worked with on a medical humanities project set out to research dementia and Alzheimer's, having recently been inspired on a care of the elderly placement. He started to talk to me about research suggesting that plaques formed by deposition of the beta-amyloid peptide had been observed in

Alzheimer's patients' brains in post-mortem analyses and this phenomenon had also been replicated in animal models. Perhaps here was the cause of dementia and its related cognitive impairment. He then went on to talk about faulty 'wiring' in the brain and how we will be able to explain all diseases some day through neurobiology. All well and good, I suggested, but what about the *experience* of a person suffering from dementia? How can we get at the quality of this experience to better understand what dementia is like? His project turned a corner and he made a beautiful film capturing the experience of dementia onset.

Phenomenology orients us to 'messy' immediate experience rather than 'clean' scientific conceptual explanation; and posits that experience is not intra-subjective or solipsistic but inter-subjective and intentional. Consciousness is not looking into a mirror within, but it is generated and tuned by the worlds we inhabit. Illness is experienced not as a unique and idiosyncratic displacement of one's 'health' but as a (dis)ordering of the way we now relate to the world.

I suggested to the student that he read some existential literature along with his neuroscience to get two sides to the picture of human existence, starting with Havi Carel's (2016) *Phenomenology of illness*. Drawing on her own experience of breathlessness, Carel describes a "transparency of bodily certainty" in health, as opposed to "an opacity of bodily doubt" in illness. Paradoxically, we may be most in touch with our bodies when we are well, and most out of touch when we are ill. Where existentialism focuses on personal existence, phenomenology orients us to how consciousness relates to others and to objects in the world. It posits a 'world-orientation' as the basic unit of analysis, and 'intentionality' as the 'glue' that binds us to whatever captures our attention and imagination in our immediate ecology. If the existential/phenomenological view were to be boiled down to a single principle, it might be that what we find important in life (and how we learn) is whatever *turns an event into an experience*.

Along with other doctors interested in medical education, what Martina Kelly fears is the gradual erosion of the direct use of the senses, particularly the demise of the physical examination. Here, again, 'warm' hands-on experience is in danger of being replaced, rather than augmented, by 'cold' evidence-based instrument-led examination. Touch in medicine goes beyond instrumental diagnostics, or better, precedes diagnostics: as comfort, reassurance and support for example – in sum, expression of humanity; but also expression of aesthetic as the beauty and form of care. When the body knows best, you can cast medicine as a sensibility rather than an instrumental practice, concerned as much with aesthetics (qualities) as ethics (professionalism) and politics (social justice).

A focus on experiences rather than events is crucial to a caring medicine that engages the affective as well as the cognitive. It brings the psychological into a medical relationship, such as the importance of the therapeutic encounter where trust is built. In such a trusting relationship, you can feel that 'the body knows best', or there is an embodied pre-reflective know-ing carried through in a gesture such as careful, caring and sensitive touch (Merleau-Ponty 2012). Such a medicine of experiences rather than events is an imaginative medicine that challenges the encroaching culture of de-fensive medicine, where doctors are afraid to touch in case patients mis-read this as provocative. This adds to our list of factors that educate for insensibility in medicine, where doctors may struggle to show 'natural' compassion that they feel has been squeezed out by rigid professionalism and codes of practice. Manoj Jain (2011), an infectious disease specialist in Memphis, suggests the simplest possible guidelines for a humane encounter with patients that can also be taken as Existentialism and Phenomenology 101: "Talk or listen, take time and touch. ... You have to be genuine; other-wise it will show". 'Genuine' is the existential part, which Jean-Paul Sartre referred to as 'good faith' (versus 'bad faith' that leads to a moral vacuum), while the phenomenological part is intentionality – not only moving out to the other in embodied acts but also allowing the other to reach out to you. Phenomenology is then co-intentionality.

The problem with this well-intentioned view, suggests Dana Corriel (2018), although she does not resort to philosophical terms, is that the in-stitutional system within which you are 'interpellated' (Althusser 2014) – or situated in a hierarchical power structure – may itself be one of bad faith: "where there, quite honestly, may not even be time in the day for emotion of any sort to materialize. Sure, you're moving through the motions, but you're also doing it all on little sleep, with poor health and hygiene, and, frankly, somewhat in a daze". Corriel continues: "Someone should really do something about that", with which I heartily concur. The answer? For Corriel: "We need more empathy in the field of medicine. And more touch. Schools need to teach it in class and residency programs need to teach it on the wards, and in clinics, instead of telling students to detach".

Orestes Gutierrez (2018) describes 'the power of touch in medicine' in terms of research evidence, walking us back to my student's inclination to understand dementia not from the viewpoint of the person suffering mem-ory loss and cognitive issues (existential dilemmas), or from the phenome-nological viewpoint of experiencing *loss* of bodily presence and embodied relationship with others and objects, but rather as withdrawal of stimulation causing biological trauma.

Babies do not thrive so well without touch – that serves to release neuro-transmitters such as endorphins, serotonin, oxycotin and dopamine acti-vating opioid receptors in the brain to act as natural painkillers. Touch also reduces levels of cortisol, a stress hormone. Children who are nourished adequately but deprived of touch, for example, in orphanages, can show chronic emotional and psychological conditions such as withdrawal and in-ability to form loving relationships. Gutierrez (ibid) tells the well-publicised story from 1995 of a pair of twins born 12 weeks prematurely and placed in separate incubators to reduce the risk of cross-infection. While one twin gained weight and made good progress, the other, smaller and weaker, encountered breathing and heart-rate issues and slipped into a critical condition. A smart nurse moved the weaker baby into her healthier sister's incubator, as the latter snuggled up to the former, wrapping her arm around the weaker sister. This healing hug sparked a miraculous recovery in the weaker baby, with blood-oxygen readings improving, and temperature and heart rate stabilising at normal. Both twins were able to eventually return home healthy thanks, perhaps, to the power of touch.

Percussion

While technologies are fast-replacing key components of the physical examination, the touch-based diagnostic methods of palpation and percussion are still taught in medical schools. Badged as 'clinical skills', palpation and percussion serve a much broader symbolic purpose – as a rite of passage and formation of identity. Medicine is processional, and such a skill set continues a tradition, positioning the medical student or offering a focus for identification. Anna Harris (2016), who trained in medicine but is now an anthropologist, has carried out participant-observer ethnographic research on the meanings of learning percussion in particular in Maastricht medical school in the Netherlands.

Situated in the wider Maastricht project 'Sonic Skills', Anna Harris's findings argue that learning percussion is not simply learning a craft, but also crafting a body, or rather, several bodies: "skilled bodies", "affected bodies" and "resonating bodies". In short, embodied learning of a clinical skill (and associated knowledge) results in the ability to enact that skill (skilled bodies); but this is also mediated by ethical and professional considerations (values and associated feeling states) within a community of practice and in association with patients (affected bodies); and finally, students learn to both shape and inhabit their bodies differently as they inhabit the bodies of their patients through diagnostic gestures (resonating bodies).

This follows the anthropologist Tim Ingold's (ibid: 40) notion of 'enskillment', where "bodies exist in a dynamic ecological arrangement with tools and the environment, and are developed through skills". For Ingold, this is the forming of an attentive body, one of close noticing through all the senses. Here, it is as if "body parts are progressively acquired" in Bruno Latour's words (Latour 2004: 207). Latour is careful to note that we should not imagine this so much as the growth of the perceiver's body, but rather the attentive embedding of the perceiver in a sensory landscape. Importantly, there is an innovative pedagogy at work here – the education of attention is dependent on inhibition of impulses based on heroic individualism (the master trope of medicine) to allow absorption into a context or environment (the basis for sociomaterial practices). Inhibition of the heroic impulse allows a set of social and collaborative gestures to emerge as embodied 'patient-centredness', a form of mutuality.

Tim Rice (2013) reminds us that such mutual sense-based learning is part of a wider 'sensory politics' in medicine, in which again disembodied technologies are displacing hands-on embodied practices. But sensory politics has a wider dimension, in which power relationships are defined through ownership of capital such as expertise in diagnostic skills, where medical students are inserted into a hierarchy. As noted above, the philosopher Louis Althusser (2014) describes how cultures 'interpellate' their members as part of identification with that culture, either active or passive acceptance of its 'ideological apparatus'. This 'insertion' affords an identity. Medical students accept the 'ideological state apparatus' of medical culture that is also, and necessarily, a 'repressive state apparatus' as it demands duty and conformity from its students until they are 'adult' enough to speak their own minds.

The material practices of medicine, such as percussion and palpation, teach students how they shall touch patients within an ethical and professional framework of non-discrimination and absence of manipulation. Touch is then riven with paradox as it follows the 'touch/don't touch' rule based on inhibition rather than excitation. A 'natural' response to touch, for example, in offering comfort, is inhibited as a 'professional' gesture. This leads to general inhibition of embodied exchange in medicine that represents another facet of the education of insensibility and the anaesthetising of social exchange.

Medical education, as I have argued, works under this paradoxical rule and regime of generalised inhibition – rather than excitation – where a body of evidence, discussed later, shows that patients generally want and benefit from touch. It may be that paradoxical inhibition of touch through clinical skills training, fear of litigation from perceived inappropriate touch (especially in intimate examinations), and a climate of political correctness (that has obvious benefits such as frustrating uninvited and inappropriate touch) is depriving patients of the kind of touch that they actually crave in a medical encounter.

Touch, of course, is not just about patients but also about medical students coming to know their own developing 'doctor-bodies'. Anna Harris (2016) notes that, while working on the bodies of patients in percussing and palpating in particular, students come to know, define and refine their bodies. While percussion involves listening, touch and proprioception (knowing where one finger is in relationship to another), it is generally assumed that touch is primary. However, it is perhaps better to frame 'hands-on' clinical skills as an inter-sensory experience. For example, Harris draws on Merleau-Ponty to suggest that learning percussion and palpation is not so much about educating the senses, but rather recognising and celebrating that the learner *is sensible*, and that sensibility can be deepened and tuned, as previous chapters have noted. I have extended this to include sensitivity as a necessary psychological component of sensibility in forming therapeutic relationships.

However, phenomenology in Harris' (ibid: 38) view has limitations in explaining embodiment in medical contexts. Phenomenology assumes a prior body, where in Harris' view, bodies are rather *"configured through practices"* or crafted by tradition and technique. This intimately involves the moulding of bodies by clinical teachers and the mastery of an associated vocabulary describing sounds produced by percussion, for example, amplified by the use of metaphors: similes or resemblances.

Thus, in the co-production of bodies and sensibilities in medical students' and doctors' use of touch in tandem with patients, aesthetic, ethical and political events are created – aesthetic because touch must be crafted and refined as an art; ethical because touch must conform to values, taste, boundaries and conventions according to patients' wishes and professional guidelines; and political because the co-production of bodies and sensibilities in the clinical consultation or bedside encounter is largely guided by the authority of the medical student or doctor as expert and holder of physical and intellectual capital in relation to patients as consumers. The area that is most fragile in such encounters is that of emotional labour: articulation and exchange of feelings or sensitivities. Here, the medical student may be more sensitive than the senior doctor and instructor, while the patient may be more sensitive than both and highly sensitised by the vulnerability that often accompanies illness.

The medical-therapeutic exchange is about two bodies remaking each other. The patient – the sick body – is the focus of the exchange and is developed through physical or psychological intervention – a drug regime, a surgical procedure, or merely a reassuring touch. However, the medical student's and the doctor's bodies too are reconfigured through every patient encounter as judgements are made about if and when to carry out a physical examination, level of confidence in palpation and percussion and developments in confidence and presence (not just how polished the performance but whether it embodies genuineness, humility and grace).

As Annemarie Mol (2002) suggests, following Maurice Merleau-Ponty, again bodies are configured through practices. Karen Barad (2003) concurs, suggesting that bodies in social exchanges, such as the doctor–patient relationship, co-produce one another. This challenges the view that persons show individual intention as an 'inside-out' process. Rather, bodies in mutual production of skills and identities are entangled in a shared environment that affords activities. The ecological perception view is that personal intention is secondary to affordance (indeed personal intention itself is both a product of, and an element in, a climate of affordance). It is whatever is afforded by the ecological context in which a clinical encounter takes place – such as a consultation or a bedside physical examination – that shapes how doctors and patients both sense and make sense. For example, as noted later, an obstetric anaesthetist administering an epidural to a pregnant woman finds that she is a 'moving target' as contractions occur. All generalised and standardised clinical skills training and practice are now refracted through this unique set of ecological affordances. How the anaes-thetist works is not an inside-out judgement based wholly on rational deci-sions but an embedding in this idiosyncratic and dynamic context to which the anaesthetist must adapt partly by protocol and rule, and partly by sense-based improvisation.

We can describe this sensory-diagnostic dynamic as a dialectical move-ment where the opposition of 'subject' (medical student) and 'object' (patient) is transcended by both doctor and patient inhabiting the situa-tional body of the 'abject', or this particular sick body as prelude to recov-ery of its meaning and potential restoration of its integrity and functioning. A metaphor for this process is intertextuality – imagine medical student and patient as two books (texts) whose covers meet in physical exchange of gesture, posture, proxemics and tone of voice. The contents of the books, however, are the physical bodies of the medical student known through ex-tensive self-percussion practice (the student's body turned inside out for self-examination and confession, regularly checked by expert tutors), and the physical body of the patient turned inside out to assess the nature and loca-tion of disease leading to symptoms. This meeting of the books' contents is an inter-leaving and promotes the development of a topographical imagina-tion intimately tied to the student's knowledge of anatomy. The anaesthetist will not proceed with the epidural until he or she has palpated the correct spinal area and visually and in imagination scanned both its revealed and hidden topographies.

Mo-Mo twins: let's stick together

Bodies are made rather than given – crafted and refined through idiosyn-cratic social practices such as medicine. Medicine treats bodies, but it also reflexively shapes its own practitioners' bodies through the dialogical acts of treatment, where touch is primary. Without patients, there is no medicine – patients may, in general, be grateful for medicine's touch, but medicine too is touched by the generosity of its patients in acting as the means by which medical students and junior doctors can progress in their learning through medical education. There is no medicine without patients, and patients are not targets in a war against disease. Rather, they are the initiators of a conver-sation that often results in an initial physical examination. Medical practice is, fundamentally, the act of translating biomedical knowledge into carefully crafted acts of looking and listening augmented by touch. Where touch fails, medicine too can fail. Even where there is no physical contact between doc-tor and patient there are metaphors of touch, such as 'reaching out'.

We are all products of touch, literally shaped by innerskin-on-outerskin. We have nine months of all encompassing touch in the womb, and when we are born, skin-to-skin touch is vital for bonding. In the first hour after birth, our temperatures, breathing and heart rates are regulated in part by skin-to-skin contact with the mother. In turn, through mutual touch, the mother produces hormones that help her to relax, and this intensive early skin contact facilitates breastfeeding (Stanford Medicine 2013). A story that went viral in 2014 was of girl twins – born to a mother in Akron Ohio – who had shared the same amniotic sac. This is a dangerous situation as the umbilical cords can get entangled. The twins survived and after birth (48 seconds apart) were holding hands. In 2017, a mother from the UK also gave birth to Monoamniotic-Monochorionic (Mo-Mo) twins – in this case two boys – who kept each other alive by holding hands in the womb, seen on a series of scans. After birth, they continued to want to hold hands. (Mo-Mo twins are very rare, around 1 in 35,000–60,000 of all pregnancies and 1% of twin pregnancies, and have a 50% survival rate.) Two years later, at the time of writing, the twins are inseparable.

Do patients want to be touched?

Toby Hillman (2014) reminds us of the relatively strange encounter with complete strangers that medicine invites:

> 'Just remove your shirt sir'. 'May I see your hands?' 'I'm just going to feel in your neck – it may be uncomfortable'. 'I'm just going to tap you on your chest'. Seriously? In what other setting could you do this without serious consequences?

Yet this is a two-way process. It is not just the doctor crossing the normal lines of social taboo to create professional intimacy with a stranger, it is the gift of the stranger's consent, the benefits of the examination and the shaping of the doctor's identity that also count. That evening, a similar set of gestures, formed not instrumentally as an examination cloaked in 'professional distance' but erotically as a prelude to sex, shapes the same doctor's identity in a completely different mould, as his or her partner's lover.

Despite the new era of politically correct care, where touch must be given only when invited, and inappropriate touch can readily lead to litigation, as noted above patients in general are happy to be touched appropriately (Cocksedge and May 2009; Khan et al. 2014). Of course, some patients such as survivors of sexual abuse or assault will not want to be touched. Carter Singh, a general practitioner, and Drew Leader, a philosopher (Singh and Leder 2012), emphasise how "medicine is diminished" if it avoids appropriate touch expressing both empathy and solidarity with the patient. Further, touch can be so readily mechanised by medicine, reduced to the purely instrumental aspects of the physical examination such as palpation and percussion enacted as routine. Here, the patient can be objectified. Further, "absent touch" – the automatic reliance on cold technologies as diagnostic instruments – can exacerbate objectification. Doctors may fear touching in case their gestures are read as inappropriate or unprofessional, crossing boundaries.

Singh and Leder (ibid) explored patients' views on touch in general practice consultations, distinguishing between essential physical examination touch and 'oiling communication' touch such as a reassuring or comforting hand on the arm or shoulder, or a handshake. They hypothesised that women patients would welcome touch more than men, and in turn would derive more reassurance from a woman doctor. They also hypothesised that touching the hand, lower arm or back would be more acceptable than the upper arm. The questionnaire study was limited to just 195 responses – 120 women and 75 men. Returns ranged across all age groups, with a small majority from the under 60s. Of male patients, 75% said they felt comforted by appropriate touch from a male General Practitioner (GP), and 77% from a female GP. Of female patients, 83% said they felt comforted by appropriate touch from a male GP, where 86% said they felt comforted by appropriate touch from a female GP. In short, 80% of patients were happy to be touched by a male GP, and 86% by a female GP.

While this is a relatively small sample, the results show overwhelmingly that patients do invite appropriate touch. Cocksedge and colleagues (2013: 283) concur, showing an almost identical profile of attitudes towards touch from patients as Singh and Leder's study above. Other factors were not isolated, such as the 14%–20% of patients who did not feel comfortable about touch in a consultation related to ethnicity, socioeconomic grouping, religious beliefs and so forth. The authors conclude:

> It seems that a large majority of our patients would be comforted by the use of touch by their GP. The demographics of the population recruited are those of a relatively socioeconomically deprived and ageing population, with relatively little ethnic diversity. If this study were to be repeated elsewhere, the results might well be different. ... touch is indeed a modality that patients feel can be an integral part of the consultation.

Cocksedge and May (2009) had previously looked at GPs' attitudes towards touch, finding that most were comfortable with touch when invited by patients, or where spontaneous touch appeared appropriate, but some GPs avoided touching patients altogether as if this were taboo (mirroring some GPs reluctance to also discuss spiritual issues with patients). There are questions to be asked about unnecessary personal boundaries set up by doctors in the face of a pervasive myth that 'patients don't like intimacy, including touch' or that 'intimacy is unprofessional'.

Toby Hillman (2014) argues that meeting patients and "gently asking them to bend to your touch" instills a set of values. Bending to the doctor's touch implies moving beyond the instrumental or functional to simply gain information: it is first and foremost a relational gesture generating trust. While medical students and doctors do need to be careful about how they touch, as noted above, research shows that patients in general invite and are grateful for appropriate physical contact (Cocksedge and May 2009;

Khan et al. 2014). It is also a political gesture of power and authority, an ethical gesture of unconditional respect and an aesthetic gesture of grace and form. Also touch is a self-reflexive gesture of embodied practice – a phenomenological and existential moment in which identity in bodily presence and authenticity in relationship are both revealed. The revelation may surprise the early career medical student who feels strangely disembodied and uncomfortable in carrying out a physical examination and may also feel inauthentic, mismanaging an impression, wearing a mask with evident discomfort.

Anaesthetics stays in touch

There are contradictions in plain sight in medicine – those who are most critical of 'touchy-feely' medicine may get closest to the body of the patient as they slit the flesh with a scalpel, explore a joint or work strenuously on replacing a hip. The patient of course is anaesthetised, but the conversation the orthopaedic surgeon is having is nevertheless highly intimate in its own way as the surgeon tunes to the relative fragility or resilience of the body part. The bodies of the patient and surgeon are co-implicated, and the surgeon who repairs or restores is constantly developing touch, shaping his or her body. Surgical instruments are further implicated in this – for example, the material at hand guides grip and pressure. As surgical instruments, particularly scalpels, have grown lighter and sharper with the development of stainless steel, the grips and movements of surgeons have adapted (Bleakley 2014).

Anaesthetists, along with radiologists, are often thought of as the doctors most distanced from the personal touch – protocol-driven and instrumental, technical and technological. But this is not the case. Anaesthetists have led the way in surgical education for teamwork and human factors, noting how poor communication is the main cause of surgical error. They are at the coalface of communication with patients – gaining consent for procedures, and reassuring (often nervous) patients prior to delivery of anaesthesia. But they are also masters of the most sophisticated of touch-based skills: delivering either an epidural or a spinal/lumbar puncture. Success in these techniques that carry risk depends upon gauging levels of resistance through proprioception. The learning curve is steep – proficiency for an epidural, for example, requires around 90 attempts, and this only leads to an 80% success rate (Vaughan et 2013).

The procedure of inserting an epidural Tuohy needle into the lumbar spine requires the operator to visualise in their mind a three-dimensional (3D) anatomical image of the bony structures and the various tissue layers from the skin, through subcutaneous fat, supraspinous and interspinous ligaments, ligamentum flavum, and then to the epidural space. Epidural needle insertion is essentially a blind procedure but utilises a well-known technique referred to as "loss of resistance" (LOR). First described by Dogliotti in 1933, LOR essentially involves identification of the epidural space by compression of either fluid or air as the epidural needle encounters the various ligaments and potential spaces of the lumbar vertebral column.

The patient's back is palpated (returning us to basic hands-on skills) and here the anaesthetist has a geographical mental map of the spinal region, with surface 'landmarks' such as the iliac crests. From this, a midline is gauged and the anaesthetist gets a picture of intervertebral spaces, between, say lumbar vertebrae 3 (L3) and 4 (L4). (Epidurals can be inserted at lumbar, thoracic or cervical levels.) A Tuohy needle is then inserted into the interspinous ligament, while a saline-filled syringe is attached to the end of the needle. The syringe is manufactured to provide the least possible resistance between the inside of the syringe and the plunger.

The anaesthetist provides a contradictory force to the plunger with the thumb that is both a downward pressure and a 'lifting off'. This may be constant or intermittent. First, the tougher and more fibrous ligamentum flavum is met, where a higher resistive force to injection is encountered demanding more pressure. But this must be subtle and not sudden. As the tip of the needle tip traverses the ligamentum flavum, the epidural space is met, a characteristic 'loss of resistance' is encountered, and saline can be injected. Such LOR here is a signature tactile and proprioceptive affordance – in James Gibson's (1950, 1979) description, what the environment offers the individual as a trigger. There is then a combination of haptic (touch) and interoceptive ('inner touch') sensation combined with a mental map of the anatomy of the spine and the overall sensation of this particular patient.

The anaesthetist both feels and visualises needle location within the various tissue layers, potential obstruction from bone and, importantly, LOR from open spaces. This finely balanced perceptual web enables successful placement of an epidural catheter. This sense-based information is itself embedded in anatomical and biochemical knowledge recovered through memory, imagination and improvisation in case of high levels of ambiguity or uncertainty, and a linguistic web of associated metaphors (as similes) – for example, in a lumbar puncture, a change in resistance is often described as a 'pop' (Hull and Rucklidge 2008).

A lumbar puncture procedure differs from an epidural insertion described above, where a smaller diameter spinal needle is inserted between the lower lumbar vertebrae and advanced to penetrate the ligamentum flavum. Here, the singular 'pop' is felt, indicating puncturing of the dura mater (the thin membrane enclosing the spinal cord and subarachnoid space forming a sac of protective cerebrospinal fluid). A sample of cerebrospinal fluid can then be taken (as this leaks out from the needle) and local anaesthetic and pain relieving drugs can be injected for anaesthesia and analgesia.

In LOR, much of the activity of administering an epidural is then counter-intuitive – as the needle enters and passes through differing tissues, so it meets resistance and then relief. The anaesthetist must then learn that inhibition of syringe use is more important than excitation. Holding back and gauging resistance is quite different from pushing through.

Haptic feedback is central to learning technique. But, again, this is not a sense-based technique that brackets out the patient. It is this patient at this moment who provides affordance for the embodied activities of the anaes-thetist. In a sense, like the 'Mo-Mo' identical twins described earlier, the anaesthetist and patient are joined in a haptic conversation, each re-making the body of the other. Further, although anaesthetic technique is generally very well established and ahead of the curve in terms of other medical tech-nologies, there is always the possibility of this context of affordance spawn-ing innovation or certainly variation in technique.

For example, in siting and administering thoracic epidurals in particular, there is an alternative approach to the one described above – the paramedian technique. The thoracic region has a steeper angulation and denser ligaments than the lumbar and cervical. This presents a problem for needle insertion and may signal back a 'false' LOR. In the paramedian technique, insertion of the needle is initially 1–2 cm lateral to the spinous process. The needle is ad-vanced perpendicularly until the lamina of the vertebra is encountered, then re-angled and advanced further. Anaesthetists describe the needle 'walking off' the lamina – an embodied metaphor (Lakoff and Johnson 1980) – to approach the ligamentum flavum. At this point, LOR kicks in.

Vaughan and colleagues (2013) note how complex these sense-based anaesthetic techniques are, making it difficult to construct adequate simu-lators for training:

> Epidural needle insertion consists of a complicated interaction of many forces: a) each tissue present has various viscosity, elasticity, density and frictional properties b) bubbles of air in saline can compress increasing compliance c) the method of insertion can vary depending upon needle inclination angle, paramedian angle, speed of insertion and twisting of the needle (torque) d) properties of the needle can vary, including the angle of the tip, tip type – side tipped or two-plane symmetric, needle gauge from 15-20G and width of the metallic walls in hollow needles vary e) plunger resistance is caused by friction on the syringe walls f) the flow of saline is restricted by the outlet of the syringe and finally, (g) the needle orifice can be obstructed with tissue reducing cutting and saline release.

Simulators, they suggest, should be modelled not on reaction or resistance forces but on the resultant pressure of the saline in the syringe. Again, the sense-based activity is paradoxical – the anaesthetist is feeling for LOR (the patient's body talking back as 'reaction force') as he or she is applying 'forward force'. The choice of language is interesting, reminding me of the poet Wallace Stevens's remarks on the world as 'force' or 'presence'. Stevens saw 'force' as a masculine impulse and 'presence' as feminine and embrac-ing. On one occasion, he describes 'the world as presence not force' and on another as 'force not presence' (Bleakley 2017).

Throughout, Vaughan and colleagues (ibid) use 'force' to describe administering an epidural, and yet it is plain that the subtleties of sensitivity and sensibility in play are closer to a bodily 'presence', a 'holding' rather than a 'forcing': metaphors in medicine matter (Bleakley 2018). Thus, a 'reaction force' in administering an epidural is described as:

> equal and opposite to the applied force and comprised of several factors; a) the cutting force required for the needle tip to pierce the tissue b) friction caused by needle shaft rubbing on the tissue c) static friction to get the stationary needle moving d) side compression force is caused by the surrounding tissues e) torque is caused by twisting of the needle and f) all of these forces vary according to depth and tissue stiffness.

Again, in terms of descriptive metaphors (and these are important because they shape both the training process and the identity of the trainee anaesthetist), we have 'cutting', 'piercing', 'friction', 'rubbing', 'torque', 'twisting' and 'stiffness'. Lakoff and Johnson's (1999) masterly work on embodied metaphors shows how language use is equivalent to both actions and perceptions – all are performative. As Wallace Stevens notes (he would, he had a brilliant poetic imagination), the oscillation between 'force' and 'presence' matters. It could mean the difference between an engaging and caring anaesthetist and a 'procedural' one maintaining a cold distance.

Epidural simulators have gradually become more sophisticated. The simplest model was devised by Leighton (1989) and has become known as the 'Greengrocer Model'. A slice of thick white bread and a banana represent the skin, subcutaneous tissue and ligamentum flavum. As the needle penetrates the layers, LOR can be felt. Finally, a balloon filled with water can be used to represent the dural layers, where its piercing represents a dural tap. While it has limitations in accurately representing human tissues, the feelings of resistance and LOR can be enjoyed by medical students as an education of the senses. Vaughan and colleagues (2013) then suggest: "This simplistic model can assist as part of a perceptual training course. However this clearly does not recreate an accurate feeling of human tissue. There is no 'bone' so the needle will penetrate through at any angle or position".

In a review of 17 manikin-based and 14 computer-based simulators for spinal injections, including paediatric simulators, Vaughan et al. (ibid) make an important observation that is, in principle, stressed throughout this book. Simulation, while getting increasingly sophisticated (even down to using 'artificial skin'), does not account for patient variation and for context. Simulation usually standardises (or has a minimal range of body types such as 'obese', 'elderly' and 'normal') and de-contextualises (although these are precisely the conditions that are addressed in efforts to provide 'authentic simulation' contexts in the work of Roger Kneebone and colleagues (Kneebone 2019; Kneebone et al. 2018) at Imperial College, University of

London, UK). It is important to palpate, and manikins do not provide adequate haptic feedback for this. And some patients, such as pregnant women in obstetric anaesthesia, are 'moving targets' particularly during labour contractions. Hence, learning through simulation in anaesthesia can paradoxically educate for partial insensibility through focus only on the 'loss of resistance' haptic and proprioceptive element of the skill, missing the idiosyncratic patient and the overall sensory context.

Touch/don't touch redux

This chapter catalogues a host of sense-based educational possibilities in teaching medical students and junior doctors in particular. I do not want to spend too much space here in refrain of the opportunities for medical humanities interventions in the undergraduate medicine and surgery curriculum in particular. Touch is the specialty of so many activities outside of medicine, especially crafts, where the exquisite is valued as much as the functional. For example, Roger Kneebone has tirelessly championed the interdisciplinary study of sense-based surgical education (feeding into his Masters programme in surgical education). Here, tailors, potters, musicians, puppeteers and other crafts experts exchange ideas and practices with surgeons and surgical educators, such as 'how do you sew?' and 'what eye-hand co-ordination is necessary for expertise and how is it developed?' (Pugh 2014).

For some time, I have run a medical humanities Special Study Unit (SSU) for the University of Exeter Medical School called 'Touch/Don't Touch'. The fourth year students study for three one-week-long blocks throughout the academic year, meeting in groups for two days in each block. At the end of the year, they mount a conference and present their work across a range of SSU topic choices. They combine creative work and artefacts such as film and sculpture with a reflective written essay. This work is assessed, where assessment is criteria-referenced. Part of the assessment is based on quality of collaboration and interaction with other students. Projects are usually based around memorable, difficult or distressing clinical encounters or medical-institutional issues. 'Touch/Don't Touch' encourages students to look at sense-based medical education and practice and issues such as the institutionalised education of insensibility, the topic of this book. Students regularly report that by being encouraged to 'think otherwise' about clinical issues, they come to surprising conclusions.

One of my students has just produced an extraordinary short film on suicide and suicide ideation using graphics. His written rationale shows how his own views on suicide changed dramatically while studying the topic, showing a shift in empathy for those contemplating suicide. Another studied endometriosis, stemming from clinical contacts with sufferers and experiences of poor understanding of their depth of experience from doctors. She wrote a series of poems to capture her empathy and identification with these women. In medical education, we should not need to 'add on' these arts- and humanities-oriented approaches; they should be integrated into clinical skills, communication skills and work-based learning (through structured briefing and debriefing). Once again, medicine is inherently an art express- ing humanity. Touch is one of its main mediums. We should exploit this po- tential and move out of instrumental thinking to embrace more imaginative clinical pedagogies.

9 "How do I look?"
Performativity and identity

Doctors' self-display in the mirror of the patient

Other chapters in this book ask the question: 'how do doctors make sense of patients' symptoms?' This chapter reverses the question to: 'how do patients make sense of doctors' self-displays?' Such self-displays of course show a range of characteristic symptoms, including: 'faking it' or dissimulation; arrogance and hubris and denial of one's own sickness, sometimes leading to exhaustion and burnout (Peterkin and Bleakley 2017). Here, I follow to the letter Michel Foucault's (1982: 351) dictum that "From the idea that the self is not given to us, I think there is only one practical consequence: we have to create ourselves as a work of art".

The public cultural imagination engages with medicine largely through television medical soap operas. Through these, and now enhanced by online searches, the public take on the roles of lay diagnosticians and prognosticians. Such modern public roles were first predicted by Nietzsche (Ahern 2010) and elaborated by Gilles Deleuze, who describes lay 'physicians of culture' as 'symptomatologists' (Stivale 1998). This role articulates and debates where culture is healthy and where it is sick, but also resists the dominance of medical authority in traditional health diagnostics. The first role is certainly not the province of medicine, asking rather that doctors join debates about symptoms of culture as engaged citizens. An example would be: does a liberal democratic society display better overall physical and mental health than a dictatorship? The second role, where citizens colonise health care, can produce good results such as online support groups for patients who are experts in their own conditions. It can also be disastrous and ill-informed, such as the 'Anti-Vaccination' populist movement (Shwetz 2019).

The doctor looks into the mirror of the patient to discover that he or she too is a member of the public and a patient, and asks, in the role of doctor 'how do I look?', a necessarily ambiguous question embracing identity, style and professional self-image, as well as a technical question embracing diagnostic method.

What does a doctor 'give off' in terms of display of professional identity, and does this make any difference to quality of care? We can think of the status-laced relationship between a doctor and her patient as, metaphorically, one of a 'Master:Slave' dialectic. The philosopher Hegel used this juxtaposition to point to a paradox of power. The Master supposedly has power or authority over the Slave, where the relationship of doctor to patient in a traditional paternalistic model is based on the doctor's technical authority exercised as prestige. However, the Master is not possible without the Slave, offering the Slave a paradoxical power. This is beautifully illustrated in Harold Pinter's 1963 film *The Servant*, directed by Joseph Losey, based on Robin Maugham's 1948 novella. James Fox plays a wealthy young Londoner (Tony) who hires a manservant (Hugo Barrett) played by Dirk Bogarde. At first, the relationship between the Master and the Servant is one of servility on the part of the manservant. When the Master introduces his girlfriend into the equation, who loathes the servant and treats him despicably, the servant introduces his 'sister' (actually his lover) into the household and gradually they play on the fact that the identity of the Master depends upon the servility of the Servant. Gradually, the Servant(s) gains the upper hand and roles are reversed.

Similarly, there is no doctor without the patient. The mirror that is the patient serves to confirm or adjust the self-display of the doctor. 'Nothing about us without us' runs a patient partnership slogan (www.bmj.com/content/354/bmj.i3883). We can utilise Hegel's Master:Slave dialectic to ask the interesting question: how will the doctor 'look' if the patient refuses patienthood? Such refusal takes many forms, for example, 'expert' patient status; noncompliance with prescribed medication or advice; lying or dissimulating during a consultation (typically, doctors always remain sceptical when they ask patients how many units of alcohol they drink in a week); engaging knowingly in risky behaviour (such as unprotected casual sex); and persons who turn the intention of medicine on its head by questioning, through their actions, medical distinctions between the 'normal' and the 'pathological'.

The last point is particularly telling. If doctors gain an identity in the mirror of the patient, and there is no doctor without patient, what happens when an individual engages in what conventional medicine clearly sees as symptom-generating behaviour, yet claims this as a form of 'health'? How do doctors 'look' when faced with a radical performance artist such as OR-LAN (she insists on capitalising her name), or Martin O'Brien, introduced in previous chapters – whose body modifications and endurance performances suspend, or place under erasure, everyday descriptions of 'illness' that normally invite medical intervention, to re-frame so-called 'illness' as 'healthy' behaviour? This might include cutting or modifying the body, acts of endurance that place the body at risk or produce pain or conscious acts of subversion/perversion embracing disgust, such as bringing up phlegm and using this as hair gel (one of Martin O'Brien's favourite performance tropes, where Martin suffers from cystic fibrosis (CF) and has regular physiotherapy to bring up excess mucus from the lungs). Such conscious, deliberate actions deny medical intervention, and then displace the authority of the

Master with a newly found freedom of the Slave grounded in resistance and transgression.

Consider a paradox concerning risk. Medicine, surgery in particular, is full of uncertainty. While outwardly medicine and surgery advertise themselves as interventions that reduce uncertainty (the ideal state is a definitive diagnosis and treatment plan), the reality is that risky behaviour is everyday. Hence the relatively high level of error recorded in medicine. Humans generally seek health (freedom from symptom) as they engage in a variety of risky and unhealthy behaviours from sexual proclivities, dangerous sports, driving cars too fast, unhealthy diets and lifestyles, excessive alcohol consumption and so forth. Whether we expose ourselves for too long in the sun risking skin cancer or suffer from anxiety and stress because of our work habits, we court illness just as we refuse it.

A stratum of body-based artists inhabits this space of paradox and generates important questions about 'how we look' to others. What is 'acceptable' management of impression and when might self-display become symptom? Can transgressive body art and performance educate the sensibilities of medical students and doctors to generate greater tolerance of difference and learn to think otherwise about 'health', 'illness' and 'wellbeing'?

How doctors 'look' – the content of this chapter – is ambiguous. It is also the ground for an identity formation. Much has changed since Michel Foucault's (1976) groundbreaking *The Birth of the Clinic* that traced the historical conditions of possibility for the emergence of modern clinical medicine and hospital-based medical education. As noted previously, Foucault characterised the identity construction of the doctor as grounded in how the doctor develops a 'look' that is at once a gaze 'at' (an overall diagnostic 'glance') and 'into' the patient's body. In parallel, the doctor's 'look' or self-presentation is part of the clinic structure that produces docile patients subject to the doctor's gaze – patients who generally fail to resist objectification (Wong 2020).

Into the legacy of this clinical 'space for looking' in which one 'looks like a doctor' (simultaneously offering a medical gaze and a medical aura) walks a disruptive influence. Art should disrupt: altering perceptions, questioning habits, interrogating values and asking us to 'think otherwise'. Martin O'Brien, on first meeting an instantly likeable and gregarious young man who holds a PhD and holds down a full-time academic post at Queen Mary University in London, as noted, suffers from CF, a genetically linked condition in which one is literally slowly drowned in one's own phlegm. While regular physiotherapy and massage clear the lungs, this is only a temporary measure. From 2013 UK figures, the median age of death of somebody suffering from CF is 31 years, although, as treatments improve, half of those born with CF today will live to at least 47 (www.cysticfibrosis.org.uk).

Martin has passed his 30th birthday and is a self-confessed 'zombie', living in the twilight zone between life and death (Rose and Tracey 2019) (www.martinobrienperformance.com). He rejects the notion of 'illness' and particularly the medical notion of 'disease' that carries the burden of stigma in the form of the 'sick role' (an unproductive member of society). Rather his CF is taken as an opportunity and a style of life. He takes up Foucault's challenge for identity construction – to turn self-forming into a serial work of art. He has turned symptom into opportunity through radical performance art, denying the doctor his or her role to provide a label ('disease') and an intervention ('medical management' in the face of an incurable illness). Martin has stripped the doctor of his or her 'look' and reversed the traditional Master:Slave roles in the image of Dirk Bogarde as the Servant-turned-Master Hugo Barrett. This is made more complex and contradictory by Martin's positive identification with consensual Bondage-Discipline/Dominance-Submission/Sado-Masochistic cultures and art practices (BDSM cultures).

Typically, Martin engages in durational art – long, physically demanding performances involving high levels of bodily stress and pain, and homoeroticism. For the purposes of my argument in this chapter, Martin's key contribution is again to turn the face of the Slave – the 'patient' – towards the Master, as doctor, and to blatantly strip the doctor of his or her gaze, now returning his gaze as Master of all that he performs. This reverses the conventional power structure and strips away the conventional narrative of medical intervention. In desperation to maintain credibility in the face of this existential reversal of fortunes, the medical establishment will predictably shift the ground of diagnosis away from the physical (CF) to the psychological or psychiatric ('that boy needs therapy!') Nothing could be further from the truth.

From 1990 to 1993, the celebrated French performance artist ORLAN (www.orlan.eu/works/photo-2/) underwent a series of surgical operations, each linked to a philosophical text, and overall asking fundamental questions about cultural ideas of 'beauty'. These operations were carried out under local anaesthetic so that ORLAN could read from texts during the performances. Her face was modified to question cultural-historical ideals of beauty including the implantation of two 'horns' on the forehead. ORLAN cleverly subverted the conventions of surgical intervention (either to provide cure or relief or to modify the body according to dictated, standard images such as in breast enhancement or labial sculpting). 'How do I look?' became the patient's (ORLAN's) question, with the attendant surgical team suspending their own desires to engage the medical gaze and to look like surgeons, anaesthetists and nurses. Indeed, they too became part of the 'theatre' of ORLAN'S performances, so that once more the Slave usurped the power of the Master.

The credibility of doctors does not just rest with their educational achievements and subsequent licences to practice but also rest with their personality and professional 'auras' – what they give off. The celebrated social commentator Walter Benjamin (2008/1936) – in *The Work of Art in the Age of Mechanical Reproduction* – famously suggested that a work of art is characterised by its originality and singularity, giving off an 'aura' or presence. (A position that was challenged by Andy Warhol's insistence that a work of art should have no traceable 'original' and only mechanical reproductions – where, ironically, the art market now seeks Warhol 'originals'.) Benjamin bemoaned the rise of mechanical reproduction that, he suggested, would kill off originality as singularity, stripping artwork of its aura. Good doctors go beyond mechanical reproduction (the inculcation of knowledge and skills necessary for good enough, or 'competent', practice) to provide an added extra – an aura of originality, invention, spark, dedication and outstanding quality of communication or presence. This aura is developed not in isolation from patients and colleagues, but as a consequence of the quality of interaction with patients and colleagues, where doctors' identities are formulated and reformulated throughout a career from medical student to senior specialist. Good doctors recognise that they are made not just by their levels of technical skill and knowledge but also by the quality of their interactions with patients and colleagues.

While technical medical capabilities informing clinical judgement must be in place, what the doctor 'gives off' in terms of display or efflorescence goes well beyond the mechanics of disease diagnosis and management. Here, we can learn from the biologist Adolf Portmann (1897–1982) who encourages us to suspend a dominant functional or instrumental biology (what is an animal display – such as 'camouflage' – 'for?') to focus on 'non-functional' self-display or 'aesthetic forming' (birds sing mainly not for territorial or mating purposes but for the sheer sake of singing – for 'pleasure' or aesthetic self-display; dolphins engage in exuberant play just for the sake of it; 90% of deep sea creatures can give off beautiful bioluminescences that cannot be 'seen' by many of their fellow creatures, which do not possess the necessary optical apparatus). What then do doctors 'give off', as 'aesthetic self-display', and is this important in the overall mix of activities constituting medical judgement and intervention (diagnosis and illness management)? Can doctors too be bioluminescent (and who is looking?), or are they generally dull and dulling as producers of insensibility?

How will medical education respond to the philosopher Alphonso Lingis' (see Alliot 2014; Staponkutė 2014) observation that our human voices are distinguishing marks of character, in terms of educating for the triadic 'sonic alignment' of (i) the physician's voice with (ii) the traditional 'voice of authority', with (iii) the patient's voice? Lingis notes the potential beauty in sonority, but where is this educated in medicine? Instead, we leave this to chance, even in the knowledge that medicine is partly a dramatic performance and involves a high degree of impression management. The rasping, controlling, grumbling and mumbling voices are left to their own devices, in spite of putting patients and colleagues off rather than drawing them in. What is a voice of tender care mixed with confidence? Doctors are formally taught to listen, but not to *speak* and not to manage their aesthetic self-displays.

The Canadian sociologist Erving Goffman (1922–82) developed a dramaturgical theory of human interaction. For Goffman, there is no distinction between 'authentic' and 'inauthentic' human behaviour as posited by Existentialists such as Jean-Paul Sartre who focus on the ethics of choice. Rather, we learn to play a variety of roles that are scripted and this includes dissimulation and deceit. We can transgress scripts and rewrite them, but possibly at the expense of 'losing face'. We are permanently juggling and reformulating how we present to others, and these speech acts and non-verbal actions constitute identities. Medical work (and the work of patients too) is again performative – heavily scripted, with typical roles, but also with room for improvisation and reinvention. Ethics do not reside in the decisions of individuals but in the scripts of total institutions, from society as a whole to the culture of a hospital. How I look in terms of impression management, as the basis to a flourishing and supportive doctor–patient relationship, is as important as how I look in terms of clinical acumen.

We can read Goffman biologically, through the eyes of Portmann, where Goffman's model asks us to see humans in terms of their 'self displays' or what they 'give off'. Appearances matter. This resonates with Portmann's biological model in its focus upon the importance of aesthetics such as non-functional animal displays (invention and reception) and camouflage (deception). Again, social exchanges are scripted performances with room for improvisation. But 'improvisation' might be 'accidental' readings of scripts, where mistakes of reading can constitute development in cultures. Styles and manners can be seen to evolve not through chance genetic mutations that may present a biological advantage, but rather through chance social expressions that spread as fashions accruing prestige. This is evident in the ways that dress codes for medical students and doctors have changed, as discussed later in this chapter.

Acuity in attending to cues and clues from others and in responding artfully to them gives social exchange an aesthetic frame. How we manage 'self-presentation' is also an ethical concern as we consider how our expressions can influence others. Professional behaviour of doctors, one might think, demands transparency, honesty, authenticity and openness. Yet here is the rather cynical view of the celebrated neurosurgeon and memoirist Henry Marsh (in Adams 2017): we "have a very complicated relationship with patients … as soon as we have any interaction with patients, we start lying. We have to. There is nothing more frightening for a patient than an anxious or doubtful doctor". In sharp contrast, the fiction writer Denis Johnson (1992) suggests, through one of his characters: " … it's always been my tendency to lie to doctors, as if good health consisted only of the ability to fool them". Recall – quoted earlier – the fictional television doctor Gregory House ('House MD') who says: "It's a basic truth of the human condition that everybody lies", and "If you can fake sincerity, you can fake pretty much anything".

Here then is impression management at play between doctor/surgeon and patient, as ethically suspect behaviour. The management of symptom is readily turned into the symptom of impression management. The art of medicine that values beauty, quality, form and presence, such as the elegance of an exchange, or its outstanding vitality or subtlety, is compromised by Marsh's overt cynicism, which alludes to a darker art learned in the clinic.

Before CP Snow's (1959) infamous 'Two Cultures' Rede Lecture, in which Snow pointed to an almost unbridgeable gap between the worlds of science and the arts/humanities, in 1945 the zoologist Julian Huxley suggested: "Art which fails to utilize the facts and ideas of science as material for inspiration, and the achievements of technology as tools for execution, is undeveloped and un-enterprising". Snow had asked for the gap to be bridged, and Huxley placed the initiative with the artist who would draw on science for inspiration, and technology for application. Medical science is a fountainhead for inspiration, but medical education needs the ideas of 'expressive' biologists such as Portmann and Huxley, and social scientists such as Goffman, to inspire clinicians to transform their clinical competence into expressive capacity. That is the aesthetic challenge. Thank goodness that we have companies such as Clod Ensemble in the UK, led by Suzy Willson, who for years have provided courses for health professionals and students (as well as public engagement programmes) led by dancers, actors and visual artists looking at features of performance (https://performingmedicine.com).

But we have seen that expression does not occur in a moral bubble: hot on the heels of the expressive are the ethical conundrums raised by performative models. Are duplicity and deceit to be accepted as part of the reality of impression management, or do we follow Existentialism in making a distinction between authenticity and inauthentic play-acting? The trouble with Henry Marsh's remark above, making it even more unacceptable morally, is that it assumes the patient is not agentic but a tabula rasa, a blank slate, awaiting impression or the orders of someone in authority. This, rather than the patient as an active agent who may up-end, catch by surprise, outwit, inform or teach the doctor as the Slave usurps the Master, captured in Denis Johnson's quote, or, as with Martin O'Brien, refuse the sick role through subversion, cultivating medical sickness as artistic capital (Wellbery 2017).

Mimicry and dress: the death of the white coat and the white coat as death

The apprenticeship system of medicine – learning on the job – demands that medical students and junior doctors come to resemble their elders and teachers through mimicry. Mostly, mimicry leads to the acquisition of good habits, but in some specialties – notoriously in dog-eat-dog surgical apprenticeships – mimicry can have unfortunate results, simply reproducing hubristic and paternalistic cultural norms where those perceived as 'weak' suffer. A typical pattern in surgical training is that young women students and trainees are more likely to be humiliated or verbally abused than their male counterparts (Ivory 2015). This has interesting parallels with the animal world. Potential prey will not eat some insects because they emit noxious substances. Other insects may mimic this as a survival strategy. Some insects also adopt the striped pattern of the wasp to signal their (fake) retaliatory powers. Might medical students and young trainees adopt the despicable and cynical behaviour of a noxious consultant in order to survive? Must they swallow the available poisons of certain specialties to be infected by skewed values? And do they start out in unthinking mimicry of the noxious only to end up becoming truly noxious themselves?

The components of doctors' self-presentation, such as expression, mimicry and camouflage, are managed within relatively strict codes of professional conduct such as dress code. Much as common sense tells you that 'first impressions' can be wrong and that getting to know somebody takes time, how a doctor appears on first meeting with a patient matters – a raft of psychological research suggests that first impressions stick, and that such impressions are made within minutes of meeting somebody (Woodward 2017). Such research also shows that if you meet somebody who makes a favourable impression upon you, you are likely to reciprocate by acting warmly towards that person. Further, doctors do not necessarily act rationally in the same way towards similar patients but – for example, in the number of tests ordered – also allow 'gut feelings' to shape clinical judgements (Trafton 2018).

Daniel Webster Cathell's 1890 *Book on the Physician Himself* suggests that doctors must pay attention to their appearance (medicine was then a male profession), recommending wearing a suit at all times and preferably sporting a silver-headed walking stick. Dress code amongst medical students and doctors has remained a controversial issue. Traditionalists argue that doctors should dress 'professionally' as a form of identification and to distinguish themselves from patients, where progressives suggest that doctors' dress should reflect the constituencies they serve and the times they are in, to include, for example, dreadlocks, piercings, tattoos and casual clothing. One in five people in the UK now have at least one tattoo. Slowly, medicine is attracting a broader ethnic mix including a Muslim population, yet covering the face for women is explicitly barred across most medical schools.

There is a movement amongst some medical students to challenge stricter dress codes for medicine on the grounds of discrimination. At the April 2018 British Medical Association's (BMA) annual medical student committee conference, Peninsula Medical School at the University of Plymouth UK raised this motion:

> This conference recognises that professional appearance guidelines are often vague and vary between organisations. Interpretation of these guidelines can result in unfair penalisation of medical students

by assessors/supervisors. (Students' dress and appearance is influenced by religion, culture, age, gender and socio-economic background.) This conference calls the BMA to:

- write clear, detailed guidelines on what constitutes professional dress, which acknowledge variation in modern social norms, with particular reference to tattoos, piercings, jewellery and hairstyle;
- lobby medical schools and trusts to acknowledge these guidelines;
- support medical students in appealing academic penalisation on the grounds of professional appearance.

A second year medical student at Leicester Medical School was barred from a dissection teaching session for inappropriate dress. He had a bright red Mohican haircut and an earring. Describing how he had little choice but to be formally 'socialised' into medical culture after some 'advice' by a senior consultant on dress code, he cut his hair short and removed the earring. He claimed it was an honest attempt at conformity and not an ironic gesture. The University of Manchester in the UK has detailed guidelines on dress code, as have many other medical schools worldwide, that include bans on wearing T-shirts with slogans, 'extreme' hairstyles, visible body art and clothing covering most of the face (hijab). (The slogan T-shirt ban is ironic as, during the junior doctors' strike in the UK, many doctors marched with provocative banners such as 'Tired Doctors Make Mistakes' – would this not be an appropriately challenging T-shirt slogan to be worn on the wards?) Women students are advised to wear 'smart' dresses at least knee length with black tights (or trousers) and plain, flat shoes. The guidelines explicitly refer to a 'uniform'. While in clinical contexts such as operating theatres, students wear scrubs. This is all advertised under the guise of practicality – you can't run for an emergency in high heels or help with a procedure if your face is covered – but of course all dress is stacked with symbolism, and such advice may, in the current climate, constitute a form of discrimination in a profession that prides itself on treating all patients in a non-discriminatory way.

In terms of Michel Foucault's (1991) analysis of the surveillance society, dress codes in medicine are an obvious point of regulation. But dress codes are also ways of managing impressions that patients form of doctors and, as the uniform white coat disappears, so too might 'selfsame' identities give way to welcome variety and difference. And so to white coats.

What a doctor wore and how this affected patients was not considered an issue until quite recently because doctors' appearances were standardised through a literal uniform. All medical students and doctors wore white coats of varying lengths (in North America, short for students, long for qualified doctors) and carried stethoscopes, or wore scrubs when in certain working situations such as the operating theatre and peri-operative environments. Indeed, across North America in particular, the white coat is still seen as the initiation symbol par excellence of entry into medical education through institutionalised 'white coat ceremonies' made famous by the non-profit Gold Foundation furthering humanism in medicine (www.gold-foundation.org). The other primary symbol, the stethoscope, has somewhat lost its functional purpose thanks to the rise of more accurate imaging technologies, but remains a potent symbol and features in impression management through the availability of a variety of brightly coloured models as well as the standard black (www.thestudentroom.co.uk/showthread.php?t=1963902). Further, nurses often wear stethoscopes.

In 2007, the UK banned long sleeved white coats on the basis that they harboured bugs, even when regularly cleaned. Hospital-based infections constitute a major patient safety issue, and white coats are often contaminated with meticillin resistant *Staphylococcus aureus* – a superbug resistant to nearly every antibiotic in use. Further, long sleeves, ties and loose long hair are also prone to carrying such superbugs. The UK insisted on rolled-up sleeves and blouses, and tied back long hair, also because exposing the arms supposedly reminds medical students and doctors to wash their hands regularly (BMA 2018a). Health care professionals are, however, the worse culprits for skipping hand-washing routines (Barzilay 2016).

Hospital acquired infections are relatively common in the USA, carrying a large financial burden, and lead to readily preventable deaths. In 2009, the American Medical Association passed a proposal to follow the lead of the UK in phasing out white coats, but doctors objected so vociferously that the proposal was dropped. As noted above, the Gold Foundation that promotes humanism in medicine runs the 'white coat ceremony' to impress upon new medical students the importance of their vocation and the place of compassion and humility within it. Other countries such as India have also refused to follow the UK's lead, guided more by symbolism than science, demonstrating just how potent impression management and self-display can be. Medical practice should be evidence-based but impression management refuses the available evidence. In the UK too, traditionalists manage to by-pass the new dress codes, men wearing bow ties, or tucking a tie in high up in the shirt. A claim is made that patients, especially the elderly, want a doctor to 'look like a doctor' (whatever that now means). However, some doctors see the need for identification with a multicultural mix of patients, for example dressing nattily but sporting dreadlocks (BMA 2018b).

How do patients want doctors to look? A 2015 systematic review of research set out "to examine the influence of physician attire on patient perceptions including trust, satisfaction and confidence" (Petrilli et al. 2015). Thirty studies met eligibility criteria. These involved the views of 11,533 patients from 14 countries and addressed a representative range of medical and surgical specialties. In 70% (21 out of 30) of the studies, it was reported that what a doctor wears does have a direct effect on patients' perceptions of that doctor. Sixty per cent (18 out of 30) of the studies showed that patients prefer doctors to wear white coats – this was, however, biased to older patients. Importantly, only three of 12 studies surveying patients *after* a clinical encounter showed that the doctors' dress affected patient perceptions. It is not therefore straightforward to claim, as traditionalists might, that patients prefer to see doctors dressed formally and in white coats. And it is not clear how patients might change their views if made aware of the potential contamination hazards of white coats.

The debate will continue – one corporate care team in America (Oak Street Health, Chicago, Illinois) describes how it decided

> … on practice-issued scrubs for the entire care team, with personalized embroidered white coats for our licensed providers. This ensures a professional, business casual appearance that may also reduce infection transmission. That the scrubs are provided by our practice is a perk for our teams.
>
> (Myers 2016)

This corporate approach smacks of nepotism. A less uptight US doctor says:

> Hey, let's get real! What about tattoos, multiple ear, nose, or lip piercings, purple hair, jeans, running shoes. In our pediatric office we had all of these, and in addition had sports team days, Halloween costumes, office decorations including hanging kites and artificial butterflies. We had Sendak T-shirts with our practice name on them. I preferred Hawaiian shirts, which are cooler than scrubs in the summer. One doc with a sparkling personality wore only T-shirts, usually with clean jeans. I think internists and family docs need to loosen up.
>
> (Ibid)

A UK woman GP trainee says:

> If I am on wards or in clinics, my wardrobe choice will automatically change and so will the type of shoes worn. I wear my spectacles more and tone down my look specifically to come across more serious and intellectual.
>
> (BMA 2018b)

This is an excellent example of impression management. A vice president for training and assessment at the Royal College of Paediatrics and Child Health notes: "Historically paediatricians have always dressed less formally. You don't want to intimidate patients or create a barrier between yourself and parents and families" (Oxtoby 2017). A consultant psychiatrist in London suggests that in his specialty clothes should be neutral, where "you want something that's safe, that's bland, that doesn't draw attention to your own individuality because it's all about the person you're talking to and you need to be presenting a 'blank screen'" (ibid).

One UK woman obstetrician and gynaecologist says she goes to work in whatever her mood dictates, and not what policy suggests: trousers, leggings, miniskirts, even shorts or sandals. Patients find her approachable and unthreatening. She says: "I don't deliberately buck the system. However, I feel that since I am not in uniform provided by my organisation, I buy my own clothes and I don't have to please anyone but myself" (BMA 2018b). Another doctor conceals his six tattoos at work, following British Medical Association (BMA) guidelines, but he suggests about doctors' self-presentation: "having tattoos, as long as they are not offensive, does not make a blind bit of difference to their skills" (ibid).

Another woman doctor argues that appealing only to older, mainstream or conservative patients misses the opportunity to appeal directly to minority groups who might find a conservative doctor threatening as part of the establishment:

> I am genderqueer, pansexual and polyamorous – I don't live my life according to what the mainstream tells me is the right or indeed only way of doing things. I don't want to be part of a profession which requires me to pretend that I am a conventional type of person just to avoid prejudiced people feeling uncomfortable because they have to deal with someone who isn't like them.
>
> (Ibid)

Maybe, she suggests cynically, doctors could wear uniforms like fire officers or policemen at the same time as they are given licence to express their individualities through hair colouring, tattoos or piercings.

Who cares, and just what cures? Does the management of impressions of the doctor matter?

One of the strangest of phenomena in medicine, while admittedly extremely rare, is the doctor who is an imposter – possessing no medical qualifications yet giving off an aura and maintaining a quasi-identity of a qualified doctor even at a high level of supposed expertise. Recently (2018), a man was convicted in Melbourne, Australia, of practicing for 10 years as a gynaecologist and fertility specialist without medical qualifications (The Straits Times 2018).

Dan Sefton – a doctor himself, and the author of the television series 'Trust Me', about an imposter doctor – says:

> As a doctor I've encountered imposters in real life – there was actually one in the department where I worked … Often they are well liked and competent! I've also met qualified doctors who are frankly dangerous. For me there's a delicious irony in the idea that the imposter doctor is better than the real thing, both clinically and with patients.
>
> (Griffiths 2005)

Sefton then meets duplicity with duplicity. I'm not sure that patients would relish such a "delicious irony". A 1996 UK study found evidence of 30 bogus doctors who had worked in the UK National Health Service – one as a GP for as long as 30 years. These cases on closer inspection reveal backgrounds that do provide some similarities with medicine. Just as Dan Sefton's fictional TV fake doctor used to be a nurse, so we find that among the 30 fake doctors is a chemist; a number of failed medical students and a paramedic (ibid).

Such cases are treated as psychiatric conditions such as 'dissociative identity disorder' or desire for grandiosity, and then medicalised rather than treated as dramaturgical quirks that may move the script on, just as gene mutations provide the basis for biological evolution. These fake doctors might have a psychiatric illness, but they were also talented – experts at impression management. As noted earlier, just as animals display efflorescent mating behaviour, territorial activity, quiet camouflage and (in the case of birds) song just for the sake of singing (serving no functional purpose such as territorial stake-out or seeking or wooing a mate), so doctors' identities are not simply grounded in their key clinical capabilities of diagnostic reasoning and disease management, but extend to wider 'self-display'.

Of course this makes sense in a variety of ways – medicine and surgery are hierarchical and 'ranks' have to be displayed; and they are territorial in terms of specialties that cannot help but compete as their sub-cultural associations demand. Most importantly, medical professionals traditionally separate themselves out from other health professionals and from the patients they treat. Much of this impression management resolves around 'non-technical' capabilities such as communication.

While researching how and what junior doctors learn on team-based ward rounds using video ethnography, I observed a junior doctor tagging along near the back of an oncology team during a bedside consultation. The oncology consultant sat at the bedside talking to the patient about potential changes in her complex drug regime. A senior nurse followed, picking up the patient's notes and drug chart from the end of the bed. She sat at another chair at the foot of the bed. In full conformity with the medical hierarchy, a registrar moved close to the consultant. The junior doctor in question followed, standing at the foot of the bed, and behind him stood two medical students. A nurse pulled the curtain around the space for privacy and moved to stand next to the senior nurse who still held the patient's notes.

Five minutes into the consultation, the junior doctor indicated to the senior nurse that he wanted to look at the drug chart and in the same instant pulled a pen out of his pocket, looking confident and efficient. She passed him the chart, which he studied for a full two or three minutes, pen hovering. He then put the pen back into his pocket and held the chart tightly, refocusing on the conversation between the patient and consultant that lasted a further five minutes. Nobody had said 'hello' to, or even properly acknowledged, the patient. Yet she seemed happy with the fulsome attention she was receiving from the consultant. The retinue waited for the consultant to say goodbye to the patient, the curtain around the bed was drawn open. The consultant walked on to the next patient and everybody else duly or dutifully followed. The junior doctor handed the drug chart back to the senior nurse and she made some notes on the chart, and on the patient's notes, hanging them back on the end of the bed and nodding to the patient as she left the bedside.

Much later in the day, I reviewed this bedside consultation with the junior doctor through videotape replay of the occasion. I asked him what he was doing and thinking when he asked the nurse for the drug chart and took the pen from his pocket. He said that the bottom line was that he really did not have a clue – he just needed to look 'in control', to give the impression that he knew what was going on. Physically taking the chart from the nurse was a tangible confirmation of his presence, but it did not signify a level of knowledge. Indeed, he realised that by this weak act of deception, he had missed a learning opportunity where he could have asked the nurse, registrar or consultant about the contents of the drug chart. In effect, the act was hollow in its consequences for the patient and for its educational value, but significant as one of management of identity for the 'doctor', as 'presentation of self'. Following Goffman again, there is no such thing as 'authentic' identity. Rather, in the dramaturgical model, life is theatre – we learn scripts and roles, rehearse them and act them out, again as 'self-display'. All was not lost – after this debrief, the junior doctor said that he certainly now knew a lot about 'impression management'!

There is a wealth of literature on historical, culture-specific pressures within medicine for medical students and junior doctors to learn how to dissimulate, particularly in not telling the truth to patients and their families in cases where such information is judged to be potentially 'harmful' or unnecessarily 'upsetting'. This cuts both ways – the medical profession shores itself up by manipulating sensitive information as it 'protects' the interests of patients and their families. Ironically, medical students learn how to communicate in their 'pre-clinical' years largely through simulated settings, working with 'actor-patients'. Read through a dramaturgical model, such educational settings of simulation are essentially the same as the world of stage and drama, where scripts are prepared for us and identities are managed accordingly. Again, read through an existential lens, such impression management is disingenuous, inauthentic, or hollow. Simone De Beauvoir and Jean-Paul Sartre famously referred to such identity mis-management as 'bad faith'. Now, we talk about 'fake news' to cover similar ground.

But the self-presentation of doctors need not be judged in moral binaries such as authentic (good) and inauthentic (bad). Recall that impression management means both managing expressions so that others (an audience) form favourable impressions of character and behaviour; or, concealing and 'smokescreening' expressions so that audiences cannot readily form an impression and then a judgement. We can take a biological or ecological view to describe impression management phenomena as showing a range of 'displays', including 'camouflage'. Many of the fake doctors referred to above got away with their identity management not just because they were good at it – albeit that 'dissociative identity disorders' are considered pathological – but because they were expert at camouflage, such as hiding away in teams, refusing to foreground themselves for scrutiny.

Camouflage

Danielle Ofri (2013: 8–9) is one of the few doctors writing auto-ethnographically who candidly faces the issue of doctors dealing with patients who disgust and repel them. Her story about disgust was introduced earlier. As a first year medical student on an emergency room placement, she tells of her encounter with a dishevelled homeless woman who gave off the "fetid smell of an unwashed body" as Ofri spotted a cockroach emerging "from a fold in her threadbare sweater". So rank was the woman's body odour that Ofri had to force back the feeling to retch. Noticing that this patient, who was in her charge, had not yet noticed the retreating medical student, Ofri hid behind the triage desk "gutlessly pretending to examine paperwork" – dissimulating, managing her temporarily spoiled identity through extemporised camouflage. A volunteer helper or aide – "an older Haitian woman" – picked up the pieces, patiently helping the patient towards a room where she could shower without a sign of repugnance.

This event can be read biologically or ecologically in terms of what Adolf Portmann (1952/1967) calls "production of form". Where display in animals is often discussed in terms of ostentatious markings or dances for territorial or mating purposes, or in terms of aggressive behaviour (such as the rearing of a snake or the teeth bearing snarl of a dog), there is the paradoxical production of form that is camouflage or disappearance into surroundings. This anti-use of the body, as meaningful withdrawal, characterises Danielle Ofri's unprofessional (by her own admission) behaviour above. Portmann (ibid: 117) describes such bodily dissolution or withdrawal into surroundings as "concealing" and "cryptic", a "disruption of the body" known technically as "somatolysis" – a strategy aiming for invisibility. It is a conscious production of absence or a cancellation of presence. It is one of the few times when you will see a doctor using silence as a strategy. A recent study confirms previous research that doctors interrupt their patients on average within 11 seconds of the start of the consultation. Even when patients were invited to frame the reasons for their visit ('how can I help you?'), they were often interrupted while answering (Ospina et al. 2019).

Returning to the topic of camouflage, withdrawal and concealment such as Ofri's – again, an absence of presence – provides a useful tactic where expectation of role outstrips current capability, a position in which very junior doctors will often find themselves. Like the doctor who pretended to do something with the drug chart as impression management, but failed then to ask productive questions, the most typical survival strategy is to avoid losing face. Further, in the face of overwhelming demands and sensations, the strategy of camouflage may tone down, dull or an-aesthetise the senses so that the potentially overwhelming bombardment of sensations that typically appear on a hospital ward for example can be filtered.

The ward environment helps with this – sharp overhead lighting creates the 'Peter Pan' effect where individuals do not cast shadows. In the animal world, shadows are an easy way for predators to spot prey and so animals camouflage themselves by staying close to the ground. Dulling the senses is linked with one of the most widely researched topics in medical education – the erosion of empathy that sets in from around Year 3 of an undergraduate medical degree and is well established by early doctoring. This again can be read as a survival strategy, much as it has unfortunate knock-on effects in terms of dulling sensitivity to patients' needs. Doctors simply cannot absorb and carry the overwhelming daily trauma and suffering they may encounter and so forms of defence must be engineered – typically developing a cultivated insensibility or dulling down. 'How do I look?' becomes 'how do I avoid looking closely at patients?'

The entanglement of stereotype, first impressions and lasting impressions produces paradoxes, as illustrated in this anecdote by a reconstructive surgeon, a woman in a male world, Lara Devgan (2018):

> An intern and I recently rounded on a patient who had been admitted to the hospital with a hand injury by the on-call reconstructive surgeon the night before. I examined her, asked her a few questions, and told her about the next steps in her care. She waited for me to finish, then turned to my intern, seven years my junior and utterly inexperienced in reconstructive surgery, and said, 'What I really want to know is what you think.' As he stumbled tentatively through his answer, I took a close look at him. Six foot three, blond, and in scrubs – he really did look like he was in charge.

But the intern at that moment just wanted to fade away into the backdrop of the ward, camouflaged, his self-presentation shattered because a patient assumed he was 'in charge' from the way that he presented himself. His appearance outperformed his knowledge. Devgan (ibid) warns that:

> First impressions do not convey enough information to evaluate a surgeon's competence. Demographics are changing. A talented surgeon may look nothing like a Norman Rockwell painting, and her education, training, and surgical skills may not come across in the first six seconds.

'How do I look?' (a plea for education of close noticing, diagnostic acumen and attendance to patients and colleagues in medical education), and 'How do I look?' as a question about impression management ('how do I come across?') are closely intertwined. We can avoid imposition of structures, codes and rules by educating medical students and junior doctors into maturation of identity as an aesthetic, ethical and political self-forming, also challenging the current trend to instrumentalise 'professionalism'. In summary, I suggest that this is a challenge for medical education to 'make sense'. As this book shows, the senses are not simply educated in medicine, but 'made' – formed and re-formed.

References

Abbey A. 2019. *Seven Signs of Life: Stories from an Intensive Care Doctor*. London: Vintage.

ACS News Service Weekly PressPac. Sniffing out cancer with improved 'electronic nose' sensors. 30 Sept 2015. Available at: www.acs.org/content/acs/en/press room/presspacs/2015/acs-presspac-september-30-2015/Sniffing-out-cancer-with-improved-electronic-nose-sensors.html. Last accessed: 13 Aug 2019.

Adams T. Interview: Henry Marsh: 'The mind-matter problem is not a problem for me, mind is matter'. *The Observer*. Sun 16 Jul 2017. Available at: www.theguardian.com/science/2017/jul/16/henry-marsh-mind-matter-not-a-problem-interview-neurosurgeon-admissions. Last accessed: 25 Aug 2019.

Agamben G. 1995. *Homo Sacer: Sovereign Power and Bare Life*. Palo Alto, CA: Stanford University Press.

Ahern DR. 2010. *Nietzsche as Cultural Physician*. University Park, PA: Pennsylvania State University Press.

Ahluwalia S. 2019. Understanding the relationship between GP education and patient outcomes. Unpublished EdD thesis, Institute of Education, University College London.

Alliot J. Alphonso Lingis, unusual character. Theater, performance, philosophy conference 2014: crossings and transfers in contemporary Anglo-American thought. 14 Jan 2014. Available at: http://tpp2014.com/alphonso-lingis-unusual-character/. Last accessed: 24 Aug 2019.

Althusser L. 2014. *On the Reproduction of Capitalism: Ideology and Ideological State Apparatuses*. London: Verso.

Amm M. Might and magic, lust and language – the eye as a metaphor in literature. *Documenta Ophthalmologica*. 2000; 101: 223–32.

Anderson P. Physicians experience highest suicide rate of any profession. Harvard University Asia Center. *Medscape*. 7 May 2018. Available at: www.medscape.com/viewarticle/896257; www.webmd.com/mental-health/news/20180508/doctors-suicide-rate-highest-of-any-profession. Last accessed: 11 Sept 2019.

Anderson RC, Fagan MJ, Sebastian J. Teaching students the art and science of physical diagnosis. *American Journal of Medicine*. 2001; 110: 419–23.

Arnheim R. 1969. *Visual Thinking*. Berkeley, CA: University of California Press.

Arsanious MN, Brown G. A novel approach to teaching electrocardiogram interpretation: Learning by drawing. *Medical Education*. 2018; 52: 559–60.

Asghar O, Alam U, Khan S, Hayat S, Malik RA. Cardiac auscultation: the past, present and future. *British Journal of Cardiology*. 2010; 17: 283–85.

Auenbrugger L. *On Percussion of the Chest*. Sapienza University of Rome. Available at: http://biochimica.bio.uniroma1.it/bauenbrf.htm. Last accessed: 25 Aug 2019.

Azari MR, Asad P, Jafari MJ, Soori H, Hosseini V. Occupational exposure of a medical school staff to formaldehyde in Tehran. *Tanaffos*. 2012; 11: 36–41.

Azer S. Learning surface anatomy: Which learning approach is effective in an integrated PBL curriculum? *Medical Teacher*. 2011; 33: 78–80.

Baim AD. Getting the picture: visual interpretation in ophthalmology residency training. *Medical Education*. 2018; 52: 816–25.

Balogh EP, Miller BT, Ball JR (eds). 2015. *Improving Diagnosis in Health Care*. Washington, DC: National Academies Press; Committee on Diagnostic Error in Health Care; Board on Health Care Services; Institute of Medicine; The National Academies of Sciences, Engineering, and Medicine.

Barad K. Posthumanist performativity: toward an understanding of how matter comes to matter. *Signs: Journal of Women in Culture and Society*. 2003; 28: 801–31.

Bardes CL, Gillers D, Herman AE. Learning to look: developing clinical observational skills at an art museum. *Medical Education*. 2001; 35: 1157–61.

Barzilay J. Doctors' hand hygiene plummets unless they know they're being watched, study finds. *ABC News*. 10 Jun 2016. Available at: https://abcnews.go.com/Health/doctors-hand-hygiene-plummets-watched-study-finds/story?id=39737505. Last accessed: 24 Aug 2019.

Basner M, Babisch W, Davis A, Brink M, Clark C, Janssen S, Stansfeld S. Auditory and non-auditory effects of noise on health. *The Lancet*. 2013; 383: 1325–32.

Basualdo C. 2018. *Giuseppe Penone: The Inner Life of Forms*. New York, NY: Rizzoli International Publications.

Bates V, Bleakley A, Goodman S (eds). 2013. *Medicine, Health and the Arts: Approaches to the Medical Humanities*. London: Routledge.

Belling C. Finding resonance: the value of indirection in a reflective exercise. *Journal of Graduate Medical Education*. 2011; 3: 580–81.

Benjamin W. 2008/1936. *The Work of Art in the Age of Mechanical Reproduction*. London: Penguin.

Benner P, Tanner C, Chesla C, Benner P. 2009. *Expertise in Nursing Practice: Caring, Clinical Judgement and Ethics* (2nd ed). Dordrecht: Springer.

Bergeron L. Rite of passage for first-year medical school students: meeting their cadavers. *Stanford Report*. 14 Sept 2005. Available at: https://news.stanford.edu/news/2005/september14/med-anatomy-091405.html. Last accessed: 28 Aug 2019.

Bernauer J, Rasmussen D (eds). 1994. *The Final Foucault*. Cambridge, MA: MIT Press.

Bernstein L. Has the stethoscope had its day? *The Guardian*. Sat 9 Jan 2016. Available at: www.theguardian.com/society/2016/jan/09/stethoscope-cardiology-doctor-outdated-auscultation. Last accessed: 13 Aug 2019.

Bijsterveld K. 2018. *Sonic Skills: Listening for Knowledge in Science, Medicine and Engineering (1920s–Present)*. London: Palgrave Macmillan.

Binka EK, Lewin LO, Gaskin PR. Small steps in impacting clinical auscultation of medical students. *Global Pediatric Health*. 2016; 3. Published online 15 Sep 2016. doi:10.1177/2333794X16669013.

Bishop JP. 2011. *The Anticipatory Corpse: Medicine, Power and the Care of the Dying*. Notre Dame, IN: University of Notre Dame Press.

Bleakley A. From reflective practice to holistic reflexivity. *Studies in Higher Education*. 1999; 4: 315–30.

Bleakley A. 2000. *The Animalizing Imagination: Totemism, Textuality and Ecocriticism*. Basingstoke: Macmillan.

Bleakley A. 2004. Doctors as connoisseurs of informational images: aesthetic and ethical self-forming through medical practice. In: J Satterthwaite, E Atkinson, W Martin (eds). *Educational Counter-Cultures: Confrontations, Images, Vision*. London: Trentham, 149–64.

Bleakley A. 2014. *Patient-Centred Medicine in Transition: The Heart of the Matter*. Dordrecht: Springer.

Bleakley A. 2015. *Medical Humanities and Medical Education: How the Humanities Can Shape Better Doctors*. London: Routledge.

Bleakley A. Force and presence in the world of medicine. *Healthcare (Basel)*. 2017; 5: 58.

Bleakley A. 2018. *Thinking with Metaphors in Medicine: The State of the Art*. London: Routledge.

Bleakley A. 2020a. Don't breathe a word: a psychoanalysis of medicine's inflations. In: A Bleakley (ed). *Routledge Handbook of the Medical Humanities*. London: Routledge, 129–35.

Bleakley A (ed). 2020b. *Routledge Handbook of the Medical Humanities*. London: Routledge.

Bleakley A, Bligh J. Who can resist Foucault? *Journal of Medicine and Philosophy*. 2009; 34: 368–83.

Bleakley A, Bligh J, Browne J. 2011. *Medical Education for the Future: Identity, Power and Location*. Dordrecht: Springer.

Bleakley A, Farrow R, Gould D, Marshall R. Making sense of clinical reasoning: judgement and the evidence of the senses. *Medical Education*. 2003a; 37: 544–52.

Bleakley A, Farrow R, Gould D, Marshall R. Learning how to see: doctors making judgements in the visual domain. *Journal of Workplace Learning*. 2003b; 15: 301–06.

Bomback A. The physical exam and the sense of smell. *New England Journal of Medicine*. 2006; 354: 327–29.

Borland C. 2006. *Preserves*. Edinburgh: Fruitmarket Gallery.

Boshuizen HPA, Schmidt HG. 1995. The development of clinical reasoning expertise. In: J Higgs, M Jones (eds). *Clinical Reasoning in the Health Professions*. Oxford: Butterwoth-Heinemann, 24–32.

Boudreau JD, Cassell EJ, Fuks A. Preparing medical students to become skilled at clinical observation. *Medical Teacher*. 2008; 30: 857–62.

Bourdieu P. 1977. *Outline of a Theory of Practice*. Cambridge: Cambridge University Press.

Boyd W. A matter of life and death: William Boyd on the rise of the surgeon-memoir. *The Guardian*. 6 May 2017. Available at: www.theguardian.com/books/2017/may/06/surgeon-writer-life-hands-william-boyd. Last accessed: 11 Sept 2019.

British Medical Association (BMA). Dress codes at work. 7 Dec 2018a. Available at: www.bma.org.uk/advice/employment/contracts/consultant-contracts/dress-codes. Last accessed: 24 Aug 2019.

British Medical Association (BMA). Dressed to impress: doctors reveal their chosen attire for work. Apr 2012, updated 7 Dec 2018b. Available at: www.bma.org.uk/news/2012/may/dressed-to-impress. Last accessed: 24 Aug 2019.

Brochet F, Dubourdieu D. Wine descriptive language supports cognitive specificity of chemical senses. *Brain and Language*. 2001; 77: 187–96.

Buck-Morss S. Aesthetics and anaesthetics: Walter Benjamin's artwork essay reconsidered. *October*. 1992; 62: 3–41.

Bynum WF, Porter R (eds). 2004. *Medicine and the Five Senses.* Cambridge: Cambridge University Press.

Cabot R. 2018/1908. *Case Teaching in Medicine: A Series of Graduated Exercises in the Differential Diagnosis, Prognosis and Treatment of Actual Cases of Disease.* London: Forgotten Books.

Camara JG, Ruszkowsk JM, Worak SR. The effect of live classical piano music on the vital signs of patients undergoing ophthalmic surgery. *Medscape Journal of Medicine.* 2008; 10: 149–153.

Campbell D. NHS prescribed record number of antidepressants last year. *The Guardian.* 29 Jun 2017. Available at: www.theguardian.com/society/2017/jun/29/nhs-prescribed-record-number-of-antidepressants-last-year. Last accessed: 1 Sept 2019.

Carel H. 2016. *Phenomenology of Illness.* Oxford: Oxford University Press.

Carper BA. Fundamental patterns of knowing. *Advances in Nursing Science.* 1978; 1: 13–23.

Casey E. 2007. *The World at a Glance.* Bloomington, IN: Indiana University Press.

Cathell DW. 1890. *Book of the Physician Himself and Things that Concern His Reputation and Success.* Philadelphia, PA: The FA Davis Co.

Cioffi J. Recognition of patients who require emergency assistance: a descriptive study. *Heart and Lung.* 2000a; 29 (Jul/Aug): 262–68.

Cioffi J. Nurses' experience of making decisions to call emergency assistance to their patients. *Journal of Advanced Nursing.* 2000b; 32: 108–14.

Cioffi J. 2002. 'What are clinical judgements?' In: C Thompson, D Dowding (eds). *Clinical Decision Making and Judgement in Nursing.* Edinburgh: Churchill-Livingstone, 47–66.

Classen C (ed). 2014. *A Cultural History of the Senses (6 Vols).* London: Bloomsbury Academic.

Cocksedge S, George B, Renwick S, Chew-Graham CA. Touch in primary care consultations: qualitative investigation of doctors' and patients' perceptions. *British Journal of General Practice.* 2013; 63: e283–90.

Cocksedge S, May C. Doctors' perceptions of personal boundaries to primary care interactions: a qualitative investigation. *Communication Medicine.* 2009; 6: 109–16.

Cooperrider DL, Whitney D. 1999. Appreciative inquiry. In: P Holman, T Devane (eds). *Collaborating for Change.* San Francisco, CA: Berrett-Koehler.

Cope A, Bezemer J, Kneebone R, Lingard L. "You see?" – Teaching and learning how to interpret visual cues during surgery. *Medical Education.* 2015; 49: 1103–16.

Corriel D. The human touch in medicine: good or bad? *KevinMD.* 17 Apr 2018. Available at: www.kevinmd.com/blog/2018/04/the-human-touch-in-medicine-good-or-bad.html. Last accessed: 24 Aug 2019.

Curtis V. 2014. *Don't Look, Don't Touch, Don't Eat.* Milton Keynes: OU Press.

Custers EJ. Thirty years of illness scripts: theoretical origins and practical applications. *Medical Teacher.* 2015; 37: 457–62.

Darwin C. 1972/1872. *The Expression of Emotions in Man and Animals.* London: John Murray.

De Lucena, da Silveira HF, de Paula LS, Ribeiro HL, da Costa Sobrinho OOP, Leal KMB, et al. The irritating effects of exposure to formaldehyde in user students of the human anatomy laboratory. *International Archives of Medicine.* 2017; 10(S.1). Available at: http://imedicalsociety.org/ojs/index.php/iam/article/view/2663. Last accessed: 11 Sept 2019.

Devgan L. Do I look like a surgeon? *#Internationalwomensday.* 8 Mar 2018. First published in: *Intima, Columbia University's Journal of Narrative Medicine.*

Intima|Field Notes|Spring 2014. https://laradevganmd.com/blog/2018/3/8/do-i-look-like-a-surgeon-internationalwomensday. Last accessed: 24 Aug 2019.

Dolev J, Friedlander L, Braverman I. Use of fine art to enhance visual diagnostic skills. *Jama*. 2001; 286: 1020–21.

Dornan T, Kelly M. 2018. Music and Medicine: being in the moment. *AMEE MedEdPublish*. 5 Sept. doi: 10.15694/mep.2018.0000197.1; Available at: www.mededpublish.org/manuscripts/1914. Last accessed: 1 Sept 2019.

Douglas M. 1966. *Purity and Danger: An Analysis of Concepts of Pollution and Taboo*. London: Routledge.

Duncan R. 2014. *The Collected Later Poems and Plays*. Berkeley, CA: University of California Press.

Eikeland H-L, Ørnes K, Finset A, Pedersen R. The physician's role and empathy – a qualitative study of third year medical students. *BMC Medical Education*. 2014; 14: 165.

Elder NC, Tobias B, Lucero-Criswell A, Goldenhar L. The art of observation: Impact of a family medicine and art museum partnership on student education. *Family Medicine*. 2006; 38: 393–98.

Elkins J. 1999. *The Domain of Images*. Ithaca, NY: Cornell University Press.

Elkins J. 2003. *Visual Studies: A Skeptical Introduction*. New York, NY: Routledge.

Engel PJH. Tacit knowledge and visual expertise in medical diagnostic reasoning: implications for medical education. *Medical Teacher*. 2008; 30: e184–88.

Engeström Y. 2008. *From Teams to Knots*. Cambridge: CUP.

Engeström Y. 2019. *Expertise in Transition: Expansive Learning in Medical Work*. Cambridge: CUP.

English T. The stethoscope: timeless tool or outdated relic? Shots. *Health News from National Public Radio*. 26 Feb 2016. Available at: www.npr.org/sections/health-shots/2016/02/26/467212821/the-stethoscope-timeless-tool-or-outdated-relic?t=1567884728577. Last accessed: 7 Sept 2019.

Finley JP. (ed). 2011. *Teaching Heart Auscultation to Health Professionals: Methods for Improving the Practice of an Ancient but Critical Skill*. Halifax, NS: Dalhousie University/Canadian Pediatric Cardiology Association. Available at: https://dalspace.library.dal.ca/handle/10222/64647. Last accessed: 1 Sept 2019.

Fish D, Coles C. 1998. *Developing Professional Judgement in Health Care: Learning through the Critical Appreciation of Practice*. Oxford: Butterworth-Heinemann.

Fonteyn M, Fisher A. Use of think aloud method to study nurses' reasoning and decision making in clinical practice settings. *Journal of Neuroscience Nursing*. 1995; 27: 124–48.

Foucault M. 1976. *The Birth of the Clinic: An Archaeology of Medical Perception*. London: Tavistock Publications Ltd.

Foucault M. 1982. On the genealogy of ethics: an overview of work in progress. In: P Rabinow (ed, 1997). *Michel Foucault: Ethics, Subjectivity and Truth. The Essential Works of Michel Foucault 1954–1984*. New York, NY: The New Press.

Foucault M. 1988. *Technologies of the Self*. Amherst, MA: University of Massachusetts Press.

Foucault M. 1990. *The Care of the Self*. London: Penguin.

Foucault M. 1991. *Discipline and Punish: The Birth of the Prison*. London: Penguin.

Fox AT, Fertleman M, Cahill P, Palmer RD. Medical slang in British hospitals. *Ethics & Behavior*. 2003; 13: 173–89.

Frankish K. Dual-process and dual-system theories of reasoning. *Philosophy Compass*. 2010; 5: 914–26.

Fredriksen S. Diseases are invisible. *Journal of Medical Ethics, Medical Humanities*. 2002; 28: 71–73.

Freshwater D. 2003. *Counselling Skills for Nurses, Midwives and Health Visitors*. Maidenhead: Open University Press.

Freshwater D, Jons CJ (eds). 2005. *Transforming Nursing through Reflective Practice*. Oxford: Blackwell.

Gaufberg E, Williams R. Reflection in a museum setting: The personal responses tour. *Journal of Graduate Medical Education*. 2011; 3: 546–49.

Gelgoot E, Caufield-Noll C, Chisolm M. Using the visual arts to teach clinical excellence. *MedEd Publish*. 2018; Available at: www.mededpublish.org/manuscripts/1749. Last accessed: 6 Dec 2019.

Ghazanfar H, Rashid S, Hussain A, Ghazanfar M, Ghazanfar A, Javaid A. Cadaveric dissection a thing of the past? The insight of consultants, fellows, and residents. *Cureus*. 2018; 10: e2418.

Ghosh S. Human cadaveric dissection: a historical account from ancient Greece to the modern era. *Anatomy and Cell Biology*. 2015; 48: 153–69.

Gibson JJ. 1950. *The Perception of the Visual World*. Oxford: Houghton Mifflin.

Gibson JJ. 1979. *The Ecological Approach to Visual Perception*. Boston, MA: Houghton Mifflin Co.

Gillespie H, Kelly M, Gormley G, King N, Gilliland D, Dornan T. How can tomorrow's doctors be more caring? A phenomenological investigation. *Medical Education*. 2018; 52: 1052–63.

Gladwell M. 2008. *Outliers: The Story of Success*. New York, NY: Little, Brown and Company.

Godeau E. Dissecting cadavers: learning anatomy or a rite of passage? *Hektoen International: A Journal of Medical Humanities*. 2009; 1 (5). Available at: http://hekint.org/2017/01/22/dissecting-cadavers-learning-anatomy-or-a-rite-of-passage/. Last accessed: 1 Sept 2019.

Godwin R. Sonic doom: how noise pollution kills thousands each year. *The Guardian*. 3 Jul 2018. Available at: www.theguardian.com/lifeandstyle/2018/jul/03/sonic-doom-noise-pollution-kills-heart-disease-diabetes. Last accessed: 18 Aug 2019.

Goodman P. 1964. *Compulsory Miseducation*. New York, NY: Horizon Press.

Graber ML, Berner ES (eds). Diagnostic error: is overconfidence the problem? *The American Journal of Medicine (Supplement)*. 2008; 121 (5A): S2–23.

Grant K. Dissection debate: why are medical schools cutting back on cadavers? *The Globe and Mail*. 27 Apr 2014. Available at: www.theglobeandmail.com/life/health-and-fitness/health/dissection-debate-why-are-medical-schools-cutting-back-on-cadavers/article18296300. Last accessed: 11 Sept 2019.

Griffiths EB. How common are imposter doctors? Here are the real-life tales behind Jodie Whittaker's new drama Trust Me. *Radio Times*. 28 Jan 2005. Available at: www.radiotimes.com/news/2018-01-05/how-common-are-imposter-doctors-here-are-the-real-life-tales-behind-jodie-whittakers-new-drama-trust-me/. Last accessed: 24 Aug 2019.

Groopman J. 2007. *How Doctors Think*. Boston, MA: Houghton Mifflin Harcourt.

Guerts K. 2003. *Culture and the Senses: Bodily Ways of Knowing in an African Community*. Oakland, CA: University of California Press.

Gurwin J, Revere KE, Niepold S, Bassett B, Mitchell R, Davidson S, DeLisser H, Binenbaum G. A randomized controlled study of art observation training to improve medical student ophthalmology skills. *Ophthalmology.* 2018; 125: 8–14.

Gutierrez O. The power of touch in medicine. Posted in: *Healing Power of Touch.* 16 Mar 2018. Available at: www.drorestesg.com/blog.php. Last accessed: 24 Aug 2019.

Ha JF, Longnecker N. Doctor-patient communication: a review. *Ochsner Journal.* 2010; 10: 38–43.

Habicht JL, Kiessling C, Winkelmann A. Bodies for anatomy education in medical schools: an overview of the sources of cadavers worldwide. *Academic Medicine.* 2018; 93: 1293–1300.

Hafferty FW. Cadaver stories and the emotional socialization of medical students. *Journal of Health and Social Behavior.* 1988; 29: 344–56.

Hafferty FW. 1991. *Into the Valley – Death and the Socialization of Medical Students.* New Haven, CT: Yale University Press.

Haidet P, Jarecke J, Yang C, Teal CR, Street RL, Stuckey H. Using jazz as a metaphor to teach improvisational communication skills. *Healthcare.* 2017; 5: 41. Available at: https://pdfs.semanticscholar.org/c4e6/1e5f8a16ff8c1c51b4caa918c3 ca3a554f7b.pdf. Last accessed: 11 Sept 2019.

Haidet P. Jazz and the 'art' of medicine: improvisation in the medical encounter. *Annals of Family Medicine.* 2007; 5: 164–69.

Hallyn F. 1993. *The Poetic Structure of the World: Copernicus and Kepler.* New York, NY: Zone Books.

Haraway D. 1994. A manifesto for cyborgs: science, technology, and socialist feminism in the 1980s. In: S Seidman (ed). *The Postmodern Turn: New Perspectives on Social Theory.* Cambridge: Cambridge University Press, 82–115.

Harris A. Listening-touch, affect and the crafting of medical bodies through percussion. *Body & Society.* 2016; 22: 31–61.

Hayashi S, Naito M, Kawata S, Qu N, Hatayama N, Hira S, Itoh M. History and future of human cadaver preservation for surgical training: from formalin to saturated salt solution method. *Anatomical Science.* 2016; 91: 1–7.

Heller-Roazen D. 2007. *The Inner Touch: Archaeology of a Sensation.* New York, NY: Zone Books.

Heron J. 1974. *Co-Counselling.* Guilford: Human Potential Research Project, University of Surrey.

Heyes CJ. 2020. *Anaesthetics of Existence: Essays on Experience at the Edge.* Durham, NC: Duke University Press.

Hillman J. 1972. An essay on pan. In: WH Roscher, J Hillman (eds). *Pan and the Nightmare: Two Essays.* Dallas, TX: Spring Publications.

Hillman T. #SoMe and #MedEd – don't forget to head for the bed. *BMJ Postgraduate Medical Journal.* Blog. 12 Oct 2014. Available at: https://blogs.bmj. com/pmj/2014/10/12/some-and-meded-dont-forget-to-head-for-the-bed/. Last accessed: 24 Aug 2019.

Hillman J, Ventura M. 1992. *We've Had a Hundred Years of Psychotherapy and the World's Getting Worse.* San Francisco, CA: Harper SanFrancisco.

Hilton SR, Slotnick HB. Proto-professionalism: how professionalisation occurs across the continuum of medical education. *Medical Education.* 2005; 39: 58–65.

Hofkins D. *From Sade to Slade: Background Music in Theatre Can Hinder Smooth Operations.* University College London, Institute of Education. 6 Aug 2018. Available at: www.ucl.ac.uk/ioe/research-projects/2018/oct/sade-slade-background-music-theatre-can-hinder-smooth-operations. Last accessed: 11 Sept 2019.

Horden P. 2016. *Music as Medicine: The History of Music Therapy Since Antiquity.* London: Routledge.

Howes D. The senses in medicine. *Culture, Medicine and Psychiatry.* 1995; 19: 125–33.

Howes D. 2003. *Sensual Relations: Engaging the Senses in Culture and Social Theory.* Ann Arbor, MI: University of Michigan Press.

Hull JZ, Rucklidge MW. Reliability of the 'pop' sign as an indicator of dural puncture. *Anaesthesia.* 2008; 63: 100.

Hume D. (1748). *An Enquiry Concerning Human Understanding.* Chapter 3. Available at: https://ebooks.adelaide.edu.au/h/hume/david/h92e/chapter12.html. Last accessed: 3 Sept 2019.

Hunter KM. 1991. *Doctors' Stories: The Narrative Structure of Medical Knowledge.* Princeton, NJ: Princeton University Press.

Huysmans J-K. 2003/1884. *Against Nature.* London: Penguin Books.

Ingold T. 1999 (revised from 1997). *From the Transmission of Representations to the Education of Attention.* University of Manchester. Available at: http://lchc.ucsd.edu/mca/Paper/ingold/ingold1.htm. Last accessed: 16 Aug 2019.

Ingold T. 2000. *The Perception of the Environment: Essays on Livelihood, Dwelling and Skill.* London: Routledge.

Ivory K. *Surgeons Take a Scalpel to their Own Toxic Culture.* Sydney Medical School, University of Sydney. 10 Sept 2015. Available at: http://theconversation.com/surgeons-take-a-scalpel-to-their-own-toxic-culture-47350. Last accessed: 24 Aug 2019.

Jacques A, Trinkley R, Stone L, Tang R. Art of analysis: A co-operative program between a museum and medicine. *Journal for Learning through the Arts.* 2012; 8: 1–9.

Jain M. Doctors often struggle to show compassion while dealing with patients. *Washington Post.* 16 May 2011. Available at: www.washingtonpost.com/national/health/doctors-often-struggle-to-show-compassion-while-dealing-with-patients/2011/05/02/AFiR8A5G_story.html. Last accessed: 11 Sept 2019.

Jasani S, Sacks N. Utilizing visual art to enhance the clinical observation skills of medical students. *Medical Teacher.* 2012; 35: e1327–31.

Jay M. 1993. *Downcast Eyes: The Denigration of Vision in Twentieth-Century French Thought.* Oakland, CA: University of California Press.

Johnson D. 1992. *Jesus' Son.* New York, NY: Farrar, Strauss & Giroux.

Jones C, Galison P (eds). 1998. *Picturing Science, Producing Art.* New York, NY: Routledge.

Kahneman P, Slovek D, Tversky A (eds). 1982. *Judgement under Uncertainty: Heuristics and Biases.* Cambridge: CUP.

Kaul S. Views from the masters: pocket ultrasound devices: time to discard the stethoscope? *Echo Research and Practice.* 2014; 1: E7–8.

Kelly B. Doctors can soon prescribe visits to Montreal Museum of Fine Arts. *Montreal Gazette.* 11 Oct 2018. Available at: https://montrealgazette.com/news/local-news/doctors-can-soon-prescribe-visits-to-montreal-museum-of-fine-arts. Last accessed: 12 Sept 2019.

Kelly M, Ellaway R, Scherpbier A, King N, Dornan T. Body pedagogics: embodied learning for the health professions. *Medical Education.* First published online prior to print, 19 June 2019. doi:10.1111/medu.13916.

Kelly MA, Nixon L, McClurg C, Scherpbier A, King N, Dornan T. Experience of touch in healthcare: a meta-ethnography across the healthcare professions. *Qualitative Health Research.* 2018; 28: 200–12.

Kelly M, Tink W, Nixon L. Keeping the human touch in medical practice. *Academic Medicine.* 2014; 89: 1314.

Kember D. 2001. *Reflective Teaching and Learning in the Health Professions.* Oxford: Blackwell Science.

Khan FH, Hanif R, Tabassum R, Qidwai W, Nanji K. Patient attitudes towards physician nonverbal behaviors during consultancy: result from a developing country. *ISRN Family Medicine.* 2014. doi:10.1155/2014/473654.

Kirklin D, Duncan J, McBride S, Hunt S, Griffin M. A cluster design controlled trial of arts-based observational skills training in primary care. *Medical Education.* 2007; 41: 395–401.

Kneebone R. Looking and seeing. *The Lancet. Perspectives in Practice.* 2019; 393: 1091. Available at: www.thelancet.com/journals/lancet/article/PIIS0140-6736(19)30507-0/fulltext Last accessed: 16 Aug 2019.

Kneebone R, Schlegel C, Spivey A. Science in hand: how art and craft can boost reproducibility. *Nature.* Books and Art. 10 Dec 2018. Available at: www.nature.com/articles/d41586-018-07676-4. Last accessed: 12 Sept 2019.

Korsmeyer C. 2011. *Savoring Disgust: The Foul and the Fair in Aesthetics.* Oxford: OUP.

Krebs S, Van Drie M. The art of stethoscope use: diagnostic listening practices of medical physicians and 'auto-doctors'. *Icon.* 2014; 20: 92–114.

Kristeva J. 1982. *Approaching Abjection, Powers of Horror.* New York, NY: Columbia University Press

Lakoff G, Johnson M. 1980. *Metaphors We Live By.* Chicago, IL: University of Chicago Press.

Lakoff G, Johnson M. 1999. *Philosophy in the Flesh: The Embodied Mind and Its Challenge to Western Thought.* New York, NY: Basic Books.

Latour B. How to talk about the body? The normative dimension of science studies. *Body & Society.* 2004; 10: 205–29.

Leighton B. A greengrocer's model of the epidural space. *Anesthesiology.* 1989; 70: 368–69.

Lerner BH. Gather 'round the cadaver'. *Slate.* 24 Apr 2009. Available at: https://slate.com/technology/2009/04/photographs-show-doctors-in-training-posing-with-cadavers.html. Last accessed: 16 Aug 2019.

Lesser C. Looking at art could help med students become better doctors. *Art Sy.* 27 Nov 27 2018. Available at: www.artsy.net/article/artsy-editorial-art-help-med-students-better-doctors. Last accessed: 12 Sept 2019.

Levin M, Cennimo D, Chen S, Lamba S. Teaching clinical reasoning to medical students: a case-based illness script worksheet approach. *AAMC MedEdPORTAL.* 26 Aug 2016. Available at: www.mededportal.org/publication/10445/. Last accessed: 16 Sept 2019.

Levine D, Bleakley A. Maximising medicine through aphorisms. *Medical Education.* 2012; 46: 153–62.

Levinson DJ, Frenkel-Brunswik, Sanford N, Adorno TW. 1950. *The Authoritarian Personality.* New York, NY: Harper and Row.

Lipworth W, Little M, Markham P, Gordon J, Kerridge I. Doctors on status and respect: a qualitative study. *J Bioethical Inquiry.* 2013. 10: 205–17.

Luesink D. Anatomy and the reconfiguration of life and death in Republican China. *The Journal of Asian Studies.* 2017; 76: 1009–34.

Macniell P. The arts and medicine: A challenging relationship. *Medical Humanities.* 2011; 37: 85–90.

Mangione SI, Nieman LZ. Cardiac auscultatory skills of internal medicine and family practice trainees. A comparison of diagnostic proficiency. *JAMA.* 1997; 278: 717–22.

March SK. W Proctor Harvey a master clinician-teacher's influence on the history of cardiovascular medicine. *Texas Heart Institute Journal.* 2002; 29: 182–92.

Marsh H. 2014. *Do No Harm: Stories of Life, Death and Brain Surgery.* London: Weidenfeld & Nicolson.

Marshall R, Bleakley A. 2017. *Rejuvenating Medical Education: Seeking Help from Homer.* Newcastle-Upon-Tyne: Cambridge Scholars Publishing.

Marwick TH, Chandrashekhar Y, Narula J. Handheld ultrasound: accurate diagnosis at a lower cost? *JACC: Cardiovascular Imaging.* 2014; 7: 1069–71.

Maslen S. Researching the senses as knowledge: a case study of learning to hear medically. *The Senses and Society.* 2015; 10: 52–70.

Maslen S. Sensory work of diagnosis: a crisis of legitimacy. *The Senses and Society.* 2016; 11: 158–76.

McDonald L. (ed) 2009. *Florence Nightingale: The Nightingale School – Collected Works of Florence Nightingale.* Waterloo: Wilfrid Laurier University Press.

McKie R. The fine art of medical diagnosis. *The Observer.* 11 Sept 2011. Available at: www.the guardian.com/artanddesign/2011/sep/11/medicine-clues-doctors-art-paintings. Last accessed: 6 Dec 2019.

McLachlan JC, de Bere SR. How we teach anatomy without cadavers *The Clinical Teacher.* 2004; 1: 49–52.

McLachlan JC, Bligh J, Bradley P, Searle J. Teaching anatomy without cadavers. *Medical Education.* 2004; 38: 418–24.

Memon I. Cadaver dissection is obsolete in medical training! A misinterpreted notion. *Medical Principles and Practice.* 2018; 27: 201–10.

Meredith MA, Clemo HR, McGinn MJ, Santen SA, DiGiovanni SR. Cadaver rounds: a comprehensive exercise that integrates clinical context into medical gross anatomy. *Academic Medicine.* 2019; 94: 828–32.

Merleau-Ponty M. 1945/1962. *Phenomenology of Perception.* London: Routledge & Kegan Paul.

Merleau-Ponty M. 2012. *The Phenomenology of Perception.* Abingdon: Routledge.

Mid Staffordshire NHS Foundation Trust Inquiry, Great Britain, Parliament and House of Commons 2010. *Return to an Address of the Honourable the House of Commons Dated 24 February 2010: Independent Inquiry into Care Provided by Mid Staffordshire NHS Foundation Trust January 2005–March 2009.* London: Stationery Office.

Migone C. Crackers. 2002. Available at: http://christofmigone.com/crackers_ottawa/. Last accessed: 11 Sept 2019.

Mind. 40 per cent of all GP appointments about mental health. Tues 5 June 2018. Available at: www.mind.org.uk/news-campaigns/news/40-per-cent-of-all-gp-appointments-about-mental-health/. Last accessed: 11 Sept 2019.

Moir Z, Overy K. The impact of cochlear implants on musical experience. In: V Bates, A Bleakley, S Goodman (eds). *Medicine, Health and the Arts.* London: Routledge, 246–63.

Mol A-M. 2002. *The Body Multiple: Ontology in Medical Practice.* Durham, NC: Duke University Press.

Moral RR, de Leonardo CG, Martnez FC, Martin DM. Medical students' attitudes toward communication skills learning: comparison between two groups with and without training. *Advances in Medical Education and Practice*. 2019; 10: 55–61.

Mukunda N, Moghbeli N, Rizzo A, Niepold S, Bassett B, DeLisser HM. Visual art instruction in medical education: a narrative review. *Med Educ Online*. 2019; 24: 1558657. Available at: www.ncbi.nlm.nih.gov/pubmed/30810510. Last accessed: 9 Dec 2019.

Mushaiqri MAL. 2015. The status of anatomy teaching in the medical schools of the Gulf Cooperation Council countries: an exploratory study. Thesis presented for the degree of Doctor of Philosophy, The University of Western Australia School of Anatomy, Physiology, and Human Biology.

Myers G. *Physician Attire and Patient Preference: Evidence-Based Guidance for Choosing a Dress Code*. Chicago, IL: NEJM Catalyst, Oak Street Health. 6 Jul 2016. Available at: https://catalyst.nejm.org/physician-attire-and-patient-preference-evidence-based-guidance-for-choosing-a-dress-code/. Last accessed: 24 Aug 2019.

Naghshineh S, Hafler JP, Miller AR, Blanco MA, Lipsitz SR, Dubroff RP, Khoshbin S, Katz JT. Formal art observation training improves medical students' visual diagnostic skills. *Journal of General and Internal Medicine*. 2008; 23: 991–7.

Neill C. 2020. Perspectives on olfaction in medical culture. In: A Bleakley (ed). *Routledge Handbook of Medical Humanities*. London: Routledge, 309–18.

Newman-Toker DE. A unified conceptual model for diagnostic errors: underdiagnosis, overdiagnosis, and misdiagnosis. *Diagnosis (Berl)*. 2014; 1: 43–48.

Newman-Toker DE, Pronovost PJ. Diagnostic errors – the next frontier for patient safety. *JAMA*. 2009; 301: 1060–62.

Nicolson M. 2004. Having the doctor's ear in nineteenth century Edinburgh. In: MM Smith (ed). *Hearing History: A Reader*. London, University of Georgia Press, 151–68.

Norman GR, Eva KW. Diagnostic error and clinical reasoning. *Medical Education*. 2010; 44: 94–100.

Norman G, Young M, Brooks L. Non-analytical models of clinical reasoning: the role of experience. *Medical Education*. 2007; 41: 1140–45.

Nussbaum M. 2001. *The Fragility of Goodness: Luck and Ethics in Greek Tragedy and Philosophy* (2nd ed). Cambridge: CUP.

Nutton V. Galen and Egypt. *Sudhoffs Arch Z Wissenschaftsgesch Beih*. 1993; 32: 11–31.

O'Brien M, MacDiarmid D (eds). 2018. *Survival of the Sickest, the art of Martin O'Brien*. London: Live Art Development Agency.

Ofri, D. (2013). *What Doctors Feel: How Emotions Affect the Practice of Medicine*. Boston, MA: Beacon Press.

Ospina NS, Phillips KA, Rodriguez-Gutierrez R, Castaneda-Guarderas A, Gionfriddo MR, Branda ME, Montori VM. Eliciting the patient's agenda-secondary analysis of recorded clinical encounters. *Journal of General Internal Medicine*. 2019; 34: 36–40.

Oxtoby K. What should medical students wear? *BMJ*. 2017; 358: j3207.

Palmer D. 2003. Professional judgement and clinical decision-making. In: D Palmer, S Kaur (eds). *Core Skills for Nurse Practitioners: A Handbook for Nurse Practitioners*. London: Whurr Publishers, 145–59.

Panayotov SV. 2017. Eye metaphors, analogies and similes within mesopotamian magico-medical texts. In: JZ Wee (ed). *The Comparable Body: Analogy and*

Metaphor in Ancient Mesopotamian, Egyptian, and Greco-Roman Medicine. Leiden: Brill, 204–46.

Peirce CS. 1931. *Collected Papers, Vol. 5.* Cambridge, MA: Harvard University Press.

Peng J, Clarkin C, Doja A. Uncovering cynicism in medical training: a qualitative analysis of medical online discussion forums. *BMJ Open.* 2018; 8: e022883.

Penner J. The illness script of sexual assault. *Journal of General Internal Medicine.* Online 1 Aug 2018. Available at: www.sgim.org/web-only/medical-humanities/the-illness-script-of-sexual-assault. Last accessed: 11 Sept 2019.

Perry M, Maffulli N, Willson S, Morrissey D. The effectiveness of arts interventions in medical education: A literature review. *Medical Education.* 2011; 45: 141–8.

Peterkin A, Bleakley A. 2017. *Staying Human during the Foundation Programme and Beyond.* Baton Rouge, LA: CRC Press.

Petrilli CM, Mack M, Petrilli JJ, Hickner A, Saint S, Chopra V. Understanding the role of physician attire on patient perceptions: a systematic review of the literature–targeting attire to improve likelihood of rapport (TAILOR). *BMJ Open.* 2015; 5: e006578.

Pick A. True or false: a heart murmur is similar to a Rocky River. *Michigan State University Just in Time Medicine.* 25 Feb 2013. Available at: www.justintimemedicine.com/CurriculumContent/p/2352. Last accessed: 11 Sept 2019.

Pinar W. 2011. *The Character of Curriculum Studies.* New York, NY: Palgrave Macmillan.

Pinar W. 2012 (revised ed). *What is Curriculum Theory?* Mahwah, NJ: Lawrence Erlbaum Associates.

Polanyi M. 1983. *The Tacit Dimension.* London: Routledge & Kegan Paul.

Polanyi M, Prosch H. 1975. *Meaning.* Chicago, IL: University of Chicago Press.

Portmann A. (1952/1967). *Animal Forms and Patterns: A Study of the Appearance of Animals.* New York, NY: Schocken Books.

Pretorius R, Lohr G, McGuigan D, et al. Art in medicine: The power of observation. 2005. Available at: www.smbs.buffalo.edu/fam-med/fles/facDevfPpt/011906.pdf. Last accessed: 9 Dec 2019.

Price-Kuehne E. Life drawing for medical students. *BMJ.* 2010; 340: c1567.

Pugh R. The doctor stitching together medicine and art. *The Guardian.* 5 Nov 2014. Available at: www.theguardian.com/society/2014/nov/05/doctor-change-view-nhs-roger-kneebone. Last accessed: 24 Aug 2019.

Puri S. The lesson of impermanence. *The New York Times.* 7 Mar 2019. Available at: www.nytimes.com/2019/03/07/well/live/palliative-care-end-of-life-death.html. Last accessed: 17 Aug 2019.

Quain R. 1883. *Quain's Dictionary of Medicine.* New York, NY: D Appleton & Co.

Quigley E. Scientists sniff out Parkinson's disease smell. *BBC Scotland News.* 18 Dec 2017. Available at: www.bbc.co.uk/news/uk-scotland-42252411. Last accessed: 13 Aug 2019.

Quigley E. Parkinson's smell test explained by science. *BBC Scotland News.* 20 Mar 2019. Available at: www.bbc.co.uk/news/uk-scotland-47627179. Last accessed: 11 Sept 2019.

Rancière J. 2006. *The Politics of Aesthetics.* London: Continuum.

Reason P. 1994. *Participation in Human Inquiry.* London: Sage.

Reber AS. 1993. *Implicit Learning and Tacit Knowledge: An Essay on the Cognitive Unconscious.* Oxford: OUP.

Regan de Bere S, Mattick K. From anatomical 'competence' to complex capability. The views and experiences of UK tutors on how we should teach anatomy to medical students. *Advances in Health Sciences Education: Theory and Practice.* 2010; 15: 573–85.

Reiser SJ. 1993. Technology and the use of the senses in twentieth-century medicine. In: WF Bynum, R Porter (eds). *Medicine and the Five Senses.* Cambridge: CUP, 268.

Rice TD. 2013. *Hearing and the Hospital: Sound, Listening, Knowledge and Experience.* Herefordshire: Sean Kingston Publishing.

Robertson P. 2016. *Soundscapes: A Musician's Journey through Life and Death.* London: Faber & Faber.

Robinson J. Aesthetic disgust? *Royal Institute of Philosophy Supplement.* 2014; 75: 51–84.

Roguin A. Rene Theophile Hyacinthe Laënnec (1781–1826): the man behind the stethoscope. *Clinical Medicine & Research.* 2006; 4: 230–35.

Roosth S. Screaming yeast: sonocytology, cytoplasmic milieus, and cellular subjectivities. *Critical Inquiry.* 2009; 35: 332–50.

Rosati CM, Koniaris LG, Molena D, Blitzer D, Su KW, Tahboub M, Vardas PN, Girardi LN, Gaudino M. Characteristics of cardiothoracic surgeons practicing at the top-ranked US institutions. *Journal of Thoracic Disease.* 2016; 8: 3232–44.

Rose B, Tracey E. Transcript: the artist who believes he's a zombie. *BBC News.* 8 Apr 2019. Available at: www.bbc.co.uk/news/disability-47852690. Last accessed: 23 Aug 2019.

Rowlands M. 2003. *Externalism: Putting Mind and World Back Together Again.* London: Routledge.

Sayani F. Jazz and the art of conversation. *CMAJ.* 2010; 182: 66–67.

Schaff PB, Isken S, Tager RM. From contemporary art to core clinical skills: Observation, interpretation, and meaning-making in a complex environment. *Academic Medicine.* 2011; 86: 1272–6.

Schleifer R, Vannatta JB. 2013. *The Chief Concern of Medicine: The Integration of the Medical Humanities and Narrative Knowledge into Medical Practices.* AnnArbor, MI: University of Michigan Press.

Schmidt HG, Boshuizen HPA. On acquiring expertise in medicine. *Educational Psychology Review.* 1993; 5: 205–21.

Schnorrenberger CC. Anatomical roots of acupuncture and Chinese medicine. *Swiss Journal of Integrative Medicine.* 2013; March 13. Available at: www.karger.com/Article/Pdf/349905. Last accessed: 11 July 2019.

Schön DA. 1990. *Educating the Reflective Practitioner: Towards a New Design for Teaching and Learning in the Professions.* Oxford: Jossey-Bass.

Schumm D, Stoltzfus M (eds). 2011. *Disability in Judaism, Christianity and Islam: Sacred Texts, Historical Traditions, and Social Analysis.* New York, NY: Palgrave Macmillan.

Schwartz H. 2011. *Making Noise: From Babel to the Big Bang & Beyond.* New York, NY: Zone Books.

Serlin D. 2010. *Imagining Illness: Public Health and Visual Culture.* Minneapolis, MN: University of Minnesota Press.

Shapiro J, Rucker L, Beck J. Training the clinical eye and mind: Using the arts to develop medical students' observational and pattern recognition skills. *Medical Education.* 2006; 40: 263–8.

Sharratt C. Why doctors think art can help cure you. *Frieze.* 15 Feb 2019. Available at: https://frieze.com/article/why-doctors-think-art-can-help-cure-you. Last accessed: 11 Sept 2019.

Shilling C. Body pedagogics: embodiment, cognition and cultural transmission. *Sociology.* 2017; 51: 1205–21.

Shwetz K. 2019. Narratives of anti-vaccination. In: A Bleakley (ed). *Routledge Handbook of the Medical Humanities.* London: Routledge, 185–91.

Sinclair I. 1997. *Making Doctors: An Institutional Apprenticeship.* London: Bloomsbury Publishing.

Singh C, Leder D. Touch in the consultation. *British Journal of General Practice.* 2012; 62: 147–48.

Snow CP. 1959. *The Rede Lecture 1959.* Available at: http://s-f-walker.org.uk/pubsebooks/2cultures/Rede-lecture-2-cultures.pdf. Last accessed: 11 Sept 2019.

Stanford Medicine. The benefits of touch for babies, parents. 2013. Available at: https://med.stanford.edu/news/all-news/2013/09/the-benefits-of-touch-for-babies-parents.html. Last accessed: 24 Aug 2019.

Stankievech C. From stethoscopes to headphones: an acoustic spatialization of subjectivity. *Leonardo Music Journal.* 2007; 17: 55–59. Available at: www.mitpressjournals.org/doi/pdf/10.1162/lmj.2007.17.55. Last accessed: 12 Sept 2019.

Staponkutė D. 2014. *Exultant Forces of Translation and the Philosophy of Travel of Alphonso Lingis.* New York, NY: Nova Science.

Stetka BS. The surgical soundtrack: the effects of music in the OR. *Medscape.* 6 Feb 2017. Available at: www.medscape.com/viewarticle/875326. Last accessed: 12 Sept 2019.

Stivale CJ. Deleuze, critical and clinical. *Symploke.* 1998; 6: 192–96.

Styron W. 1992. *Darkness Visible.* London Vintage.

Sugata Y, Miyaso H, Odaka Y, Komiyama M, Sakamoto N, Mori C, Matsuno Y. Levels of formaldehyde vapor released from embalmed cadavers in each dissection stage. *Environmental Science and Pollution Research International.* 2016; 23: 16176–82. Available at: www.ncbi.nlm.nih.gov/pmc/articles/PMC4975760/. Last accessed: 12 Sept 2019.

Süskind P. 1986. *Perfume: The Story of a Murderer.* New York, NY: Vintage International.

The Straits Times. Fake gynaecologist in Australia jailed for years of fraud and assault on patients. 6 Jul 2018. Available at: www.straitstimes.com/asia/australianz/fake-gynaecologist-in-australia-jailed-for-years-of-assault-and-fraud-on-patients. Last accessed: 24 Aug 2019

Thompson C, Dowding D. 2002. *Clinical Decision Making and Judgement in Nursing.* Edinburgh: Churchill-Livingstone.

Trafton A. Doctors rely on more than just data for medical decision-making. *Science Daily.* 20 Jul 2018. Available at: www.sciencedaily.com/releases/2018/07/180720112823.htm. Last accessed: 24 Aug 2019.

Uono S, Hietanen JK. Eye contact perception in the west and east: a cross-cultural study. *PLoS ONE.* 2015; 10: e0118094. doi: 10.1371/journal.pone.0118094. Last accessed: 12 Sept 2019.

Ursitti C. The phenomenology of olfactory perception: an interview with Cara Ursitti. *Art and Research.* 2008; 2 (Summer). Available at: www.artandresearch.org.uk/v2n1/ursitti.html. Last accessed: 12 Sept 2019.

Vahed N, Kabiri N, Oskouei MM, et al. The effect of music in operating room: a systematic review. *BMJ Open*. 2016; 7: Suppl 1. Available at: https://bmjopen. bmj.com/content/7/Suppl_1/bmjopen-2016-015415.130. Last accessed: 13 Sept 2019.

Van der Niet A. When I say ... affordance perception. *Medical Education*. 2018; 52: 362–63.

Vannini P, Waskul DD, Gottschalk S, Rambo C. Sound acts: elocution, somatic work, and the performance of sonic alignment. *Journal of Contemporary Ethnography*. 2010; 39: 328–53.

Vaughan N, Dubey VN, Wee MY, Isaacs R. Towards a realistic in vitro experience of epidural Tuohy needle insertion. *Proceedings of the Institution of Mechanical Engineers, Part H*. 2013; 227: 767–77.

Verghese A. 1994. *My Own Country: A Doctor's Story of a Town and its People in the Age of AIDS*. New York, NY: Simon & Schuster.

Verghese A. 1999. *The Tennis Partner*. London: Vintage.

Verghese A. 2010. *Cutting for Stone*. London: Chatto & Windus.

Verghese A, Brady E, Kapur CC, Horwitz RI. The bedside evaluation: ritual and reason. *Annals of Internal Medicine*. 2011; 155: 550–53.

Vize E. The sound of surgery. *Scope*. 8 Mar 2010. Available at: http://medscope. blogspot.com/2010/03/sound-of-surgery.html. Last accessed: 13 Sept 2019.

Vukanovic-Criley JM, Criley S, Warde CM, Boker JR, Guevara-Matheus L, Churchill WH, Nelson WP, Criley JM. Competency in cardiac examination skills in medical students, trainees, physicians, and faculty: a multicenter study. *Archives of Internal Medicine*. 2006; 166: 610–16.

Warner JH, Edmonson J. 2009. *Dissection: Photographs of a Rite of Passage in American Medicine 1880–1930*. Jackson, TN: Blast Books.

Welch GH, Schwartz LM, Woloshin S. 2011. *Over-Diagnosed: Making People Sick in the Pursuit of Health*. Boston, MA: Beacon Press.

Weldon SM, Korkiakangas T, Kneebone R. How simulation techniques and approaches can be used to compare, contrast and improve care: an immersive simulation of a three-Michelin star restaurant and a day surgery unit. *BMJ Simulation & Technology Enhanced Learning*. 2019. doi: 10.1136/bmjstel-2018-000433. Last accessed: 13 Sept 2019.

Wellbery C. 2017. How to see pain. In: A Bleakley, L Lynch, G Whelan (eds). *Risk and Regulation at the Interface of Medicine and the Arts: Dangerous Currents*. Newcastle-Upon-Tyne: Cambridge Scholars Publishing, 74–80.

Wellbery C, McAteer R. The art of observation: a pedagogical framework. *Academic Medicine*. 2015; 90: 1624–30.

Wiens JA. Spatial scaling in ecology. *Functional Ecology*. 1989; 3: 385–97.

Williams I. 2014. *The Bad Doctor*. Oxford: Myriad.

Williams I. 2019. *The Lady Doctor*. Oxford: Myriad.

Wong J. 2020. Hospitaland. In: A Bleakley (ed). *Routledge Handbook of the Medical Humanities*. London: Routledge, 123–26.

Woodward M. The psychology of a first impression: three tips for making a good one. *Psychology Today*. 9 May 2017. Available at: www.psychologytoday.com/ gb/blog/spotting-opportunity/201705/the-psychology-first-impression. Last accessed: 24 Aug 2019.

Woywodt A, Herrmann A, Kielstein JT, Haller H, Haubitz M, Purnhagen H. A novel multimedia tool to improve bedside teaching of cardiac auscultation. *BMJ*

Postgraduate Medical Journal 2004; 80 (944). Available at: https://pmj.bmj.com/content/80/944/355.full. Last accessed: 22 Sept 2019.

Yates F. 1966. *The Art of Memory*. London: Bodley Head.

Young K. Disembodiment: the phenomenology of the body in medical examinations. *Semiotica*. 1989; 73: 43–66.

Zhou S. To medical students: we're all in the same boat. *KevinMD*. 4 May 2014. Available at: www.kevinmd.com/blog/2014/05/medical-students-boat.html. Last accessed: 13 Aug 2019.

Index

Printed in the United States
by Baker & Taylor Publisher Services